More Praise for *Mind Your Heart*

"*Mind Your Heart* is the perfect blend of up-to-date science and timeless practical advice. I wish more of my physician colleagues were familiar with this book's tactics for lowering risk of heart disease through the mind-heart connection. I intend to keep this book handy to help teach my patients some of the simple tools for reducing stress—and to use a few of them myself."

—Thomas H. Lee, M.D., Medical Director,
Partners Community HealthCare, Inc.;
Editor in Chief, *Harvard Health Letter*

"Coronary heart disease is the leading cause of death and disability in the United States today, and it will continue to be for the foreseeable future. This is true despite the fact that *existing knowledge* provides us with enough information to prevent the vast majority of coronary heart disease events in our society. Optimal prevention can only be accomplished by a true partnership between patients and their caregivers. *Mind Your Heart* is an absolutely terrific bridge to help make that happen. It presents a thorough and strikingly clear approach, explained by wonderful partners—an experienced nurse and internationally renowned physician who truly know how to approach patients and how to help them make important changes. Every patient who has heart disease, or might have heart disease, should read this book."

—Richard C. Pasternak, M.D., Director of Preventive Cardiology
and Cardiac Rehabilitation, Massachusetts General Hospital

"For people who want to be heart-healthy but feel bombarded by confusing messages from the press and from doctors, this book explains how to adopt a healthier life-style—and enjoy it. It will be useful for people who've developed heart disease, and even more useful for people who don't have heart disease and want to reduce their chances of ever getting it."

—Richard T. Lee, M.D., Associate Professor of Medicine,
Harvard Medical School, Massachusetts Institute of Technology,
and Brigham and Women's Hospital

Harvard Medical School Family Health Guide by the Harvard Medical
  School
Six Steps to Increased Fertility by Robert L. Barbieri, M.D., Alice
  D. Domar, Ph.D., and Kevin R. Loughlin, M.D.
The Arthritis Action Program by Michael E. Weinblatt, M.D.
Healthy Women, Healthy Lives by Susan E. Hankinson, Sc.D.,
  Graham A. Colditz, M.D., Dr. PH., JoAnn E. Manson, M.D.,
  and Frank E. Speizer, M.D.
Eat, Drink, and Be Healthy by Walter C. Willett, M.D.
The Aging Eye by the Harvard Medical School
The Sensitive Gut by the Harvard Medical School
The Harvard Medical School Guide to Men's Health by Harvey B.
  Simon, M.D.
The Harvard Medical School Guide to Taking Control of Asthma by
  Christopher H. Fanta, M.D., Lynda M. Cristiano, M.D., Kenan
  E. Haver, M.D., with Nancy Waring, Ph.D.
Mind Over Menopause by Leslee Kagan, M.S., N.P., Bruce Kessel,
  M.D., and Herbert Benson, M.D.

Mind Your Heart

A Mind/Body Approach to Stress Management,

Exercise, and Nutrition for Heart Health

Aggie Casey, M.S., R.N.

Herbert Benson, M.D.

with Ann MacDonald

FREE PRESS

New York   London   Toronto   Sydney

*f*P

FREE PRESS
A Division of Simon & Schuster, Inc.
1230 Avenue of the Americas
New York, NY 10020

First Free Press trade paperback edition 2004

FREE PRESS and colophon are trademarks
of Simon & Schuster, Inc.

For information regarding special discounts for bulk purchases,
please contact Simon & Schuster Special Sales at
1-800-456-6798 or business@simonandschuster.com

Manufactured in the United States of America

10   9   8   7   6   5   4   3   2   1

Library of Congress Cataloging-in-Publication Data

Casey, Aggie.
   Mind your heart : a mind/body approach to stress management, exercise, and nutrition for
heart health / Aggie Casey, Herbert Benson, with Ann MacDonald.
      p.   cm.
   Includes index.
   1. Health.   2. Mind and body.   3. Heart—Diseases—Prevention.   4. Exercise.
5. Nutrition.   I. Benson, Herbert.   II. MacDonald, Ann.   III. Title.

   RA776.C353   2004
   613'.0434—dc22   2003049463

   ISBN 0-7432-3702-1

To Ali

To Marilyn

And to all our patients, from whom we've learned so much.

THE IDEAS AND ADVICE offered in these pages reflect the integrated approach to patient care that we practice at the Mind/Body Medical Institute. We would like to acknowledge all of our colleagues at the Mind/Body Medical Institute for their pioneering work in the field of mind/body medicine and thank them for sharing their knowledge and experiences with us. We would especially like to thank our colleagues in the Cardiac Wellness Program, Jim Huddleston, AnnMarie White, Marc O'Meara, and Sarah Lynch. Their enthusiasm and support made this book a reality. Special thanks go to Marc O'Meara for his expertise in writing the nutrition chapters and to Jim Huddleston for writing the exercise chapter and for his thoughtful and thorough editing of our initial manuscript.

We offer warm thanks to Ann MacDonald for her guidance and tireless effort in searching the medical literature and helping to write this book. We are also indebted to Alice D. Domar, Ph.D., for her insightful comments about this manuscript. In addition, we would like to thank our colleagues at Harvard Medical School for helping to make this book a reality. Anthony Komaroff, M.D., editor in chief at Harvard Health Publications, provided invaluable editorial guidance while we wrote. Edward Coburn, publishing director, and Joan McGrath, editorial coordinator, provided encouragement, resources, and—most important—kept us focused on the readers' needs.

We would like to thank Bill Rosen, vice president and executive editor at Free Press, for launching this series from Harvard Medical School. Andrea Au was an invaluable editor whose careful reading and helpful comments improved our manuscript immensely. Special thanks to copy editor Jason Warshof and production editor Jonathon Brodman.

To our families:

I, Aggie Casey, would like to thank my husband, Charlie Barros, for his love and support during the past fourteen years, and my daughter, Ali, for the joy she brings to my life every day.

I, Herbert Benson, am forever grateful to my wife, Marilyn.

Finally, we would like to thank our patients for their willingness to share their stories and for allowing us to be part of their journey toward heart health.

Aggie Casey, M.S., R.N.
Herbert Benson, M.D.

Contents

Mind Your Heart

Congratulations! By picking up this book, you have taken the first step toward improving the health of your heart.

As health care professionals, we see people every day who are concerned about heart disease. Perhaps, like some of our patients, you are recovering from a heart attack or have experienced chest pain known as angina. You may be concerned that you are at risk for a heart attack or stroke because you have high blood pressure, diabetes, or high cholesterol. If so, we think this book will provide helpful advice about how you can make changes, starting today, that will improve the health of your heart.

Mind Your Heart builds on the authors' more than thirty-five years of research and patient care. Here you will find, for the first time, a step-by-step guide to heart health that combines the latest information about stress management, nutrition, and exercise. This complements advice offered in earlier books by Dr. Herbert Benson, especially *The Relaxation Response* and *The Wellness Book*.

The strategies we describe in these pages are the same ones that we offer to patients in our Cardiac Wellness Program at the Mind/Body Medical Institute. The basic Cardiac Wellness Program lasts for thirteen consecutive weeks, during which participants attend weekly three-hour sessions. The Extended Cardiac Wellness Program lasts for twelve months and consists of thirteen weekly three-hour sessions and eighteen bimonthly three-hour sessions. Many of our patients are referred to the clinic after being diagnosed with heart disease. Slightly more than half of our patients are men. Ages vary, but most people are between fifty-five and sixty years old when they enter our program.

The Cardiac Wellness Program is just one of several clinical programs that we offer at the Mind/Body Medical Institute. We also run programs to help people deal with infertility, insomnia, menopause, chronic pain, and general stress-related symptoms. Founded in 1988 at Beth Israel Deaconess Medical Center, in Boston, the Mind/Body Medical Institute is a nonprofit organization dedicated to advancing scientific research, public education, and professional training in the field of behavioral medicine. This field, also known as mind/body medicine, aims to foster your own natural capacity to heal in a way that enhances more traditional medical approaches such as medication and surgery. At the Mind/Body Medical Institute, we employ an interdisciplinary team of exercise physiologists, advanced practice nurses, dietitians, psychologists, and physicians who together have developed the techniques you will find in this book.

Of course, we realize that it is not easy to make changes in behavior and lifestyle. We also respect the fact that you are an individual. For both these reasons, we've included quizzes and exercises to help you identify your own particular risks as well as a number of strategies and techniques for behavior change, so that you can choose the ones you feel most comfortable with.

Thousands of people have already completed our mind/body programs and made significant changes in their lives. We hope that this book will provide a useful road map for you as you embark on your own journey of change. Happy reading!

Aggie Casey, M.S., R.N.
Herbert Benson, M.D.

Chapter 1

Mind Your Heart

I F YOU HAVE HEART DISEASE, you are not alone. An astounding one in five people in this country has already suffered a heart attack or stroke, or has high blood pressure. One in two men, and one in three women, can expect to develop heart disease after age forty.

Fortunately, heart disease is largely preventable. By changing certain behaviors, you can significantly reduce your risk of developing heart disease or improve your chance of recovery if you've already had a heart attack. The game plan is deceptively simple: stop smoking, eat better, exercise regularly, and reduce stress. By following these steps, you will counter the major factors that put you at risk in the first place. And it's never too late—or too early—to start. No matter what your age, adopting healthy habits can significantly improve the health of your heart.

Of course, changing behaviors and habits—and then maintaining that change—is notoriously difficult. That is why our goal is to help you become more mindful of situations and behaviors that put you at risk, and then help you develop your own individual strategy for healthy change.

The advice we offer in this book should supplement any advice you receive from your primary care physician and other health care providers. Our intent is not to provide an alternative approach but one that complements traditional medicine. Although we encourage you to use the quizzes and exercises in this book to help you play a more active role in your health care, we also expect that you will continue to see your health care providers on a regular basis for medical care and checkups.

SIDEBAR 1

HEART DISEASE: THE NATION'S LEADING KILLER

- Almost 61 million Americans suffer from at least one form of cardiovascular disease.
- 50 million have high blood pressure
- 7 million have suffered a heart attack
- 4½ million have experienced a stroke
- Every year, two out of every five deaths are caused by heart disease.
- Heart disease kills more people than the next six leading causes of death (including cancer and accidents) combined.
- Men are at greater risk than women of dying of a coronary event before age sixty, but afterward heart disease is an equal opportunity killer.
- One in ten women between ages forty-five and sixty-four has heart disease; after age sixty-five, the rate increases to one in four.

■ The Three-Legged Stool

The advice we offer in this book is the same as what we provide to patients in our Cardiac Wellness Program. Like all the programs we offer through the Mind/Body Medical Institute, the Cardiac Wellness Program is based on the philosophy that optimal health care resem-

bles a three-legged stool. One leg of the stool consists of medication. A second represents surgical intervention. The third signi-
fies self-care, the strategies you employ to enhance your own
natural capacity to heal. This third leg includes many of the techniques we'll discuss later on: the relaxation response, exercise,
nutrition, and cognitive approaches (changing the way you think).
Though all three legs of the stool have been validated through scientific research, all too often patients and physicians ignore the
self-care leg. Disregarding self-care can result in a health care approach that is as wobbly and off-balance as, well, a two-legged
stool.

Our goal in this book is to offer a more balanced approach. Not
only will we address the physical aspects of your illness—in this
case, heart disease—but we also hope to change the types of attitudes and behaviors that may be contributing to your symptoms.
In the pages that follow, you will learn more about the various factors that increase your risk for heart disease and how to reduce
that risk. Some, such as high blood pressure and cholesterol, will
sound familiar. We'll discuss the latest research findings and describe current medical and surgical treatments. But we'll spend
most of our time discussing risk factors for heart disease, such as
stress, depression, anger, hostility, decreased social support, physical inactivity, and poor nutrition.

We'll provide strategies to help you reduce stress and elicit the
healing relaxation response. You will learn how to exercise to improve your heart health and how to prepare more nutritious
meals. We also hope to help you discover how to become more
mindful of the world around you and to view life in a more positive way.

These strategies are all based on the premise that mind and
body are inextricably linked. You probably know about the mind/
body connection instinctively. Have you ever been embarrassed by
something and felt your face flush? Have you ever found yourself
stuck in traffic and become so angry that your heart beats fast and

you breathe in short, quick bursts? Have you ever looked at a big piece of chocolate cake and felt your mouth water? Or felt your mood improve after taking a brisk walk on a sunny day? These are all examples of the mind/body connection at work.

SIDEBAR 2

HOW HEART SMART ARE YOU?

How knowledgeable are you about heart disease? Take this short quiz and find out. Answers are printed at the bottom.

1. Which of the following put(s) you at risk for heart disease?
   a. Smoking
   b. High blood pressure
   c. Sedentary lifestyle
   d. All of the above

2. What is the leading dietary cause of elevated blood cholesterol?
   a. Eating too many foods that are high in cholesterol (such as eggs)
   b. Eating too many foods that are high in saturated fats and trans fats (such as red meat or fast-food)

3. Which of the following psychosocial factors contributes to heart disease? Pick all that apply.
   a. Hostility and anger
   b. Happy-go-lucky attitude
   c. Depression

4. What type of stress is more damaging to the heart?
   a. A major stress, such as losing a job
   b. Accumulation of minor stresses, such as getting stuck in traffic or being late for an appointment

5. What is the best type of aerobic exercise for your heart?
   a. Moderate-intensity walking
   b. Swimming
   c. Riding a bicycle
   d. Any physical activity you enjoy

ANSWERS:
1. d—All of the above.
2. b—Recent research shows that foods high in saturated fats and trans fats contribute more to high levels of blood cholesterol than do foods such as eggs and liver, which actually contain cholesterol.
3. a and c—We used to think that type A personalities were at greatest risk, but it turns out that a subtype of type A, involving negative emotions such as hostility and anger, is much more to blame. Recent research has shown that depression may be an even more significant risk factor.
4. b—The accumulation of minor stresses actually takes more of a toll on the heart.
5. d—All types of aerobic exercise are good for your heart, so choose the one you like.

■ The Mind/Body Link

Mind/body medicine got its start in the late 1960s when researchers (including one of us, Dr. Herbert Benson) provided the first convincing evidence that it was possible to calm the body simply by quieting the mind. At the time, Dr. Benson was working with colleagues at Harvard Medical School to determine the causes and effects of high blood pressure. The researchers were conducting biofeedback experiments in monkeys to see if various rewards would raise or lower blood pressure and if punishment (which increased stress on the monkeys) would raise it. Several practitioners of transcendental meditation learned of Dr. Benson's work on stress and hypertension and visited him. They claimed that they could lower their own blood pressure by meditating.

The concept intrigued Dr. Benson, but he knew most of his Harvard colleagues would be skeptical. At the time, few believed that a link existed between stress and high blood pressure. But the meditation practitioners persisted, visiting Dr. Benson repeatedly. He finally agreed to take a series of physiological measurements to determine the effects of meditation on the body. As it happened, a separate team in California, led by Drs. Robert Keith Wallace and Archie F. Wilson, were simultaneously conducting related experiments. Both teams of researchers reached similar conclusions based on the physiological readings, and these findings have been confirmed and expanded in subsequent research: Meditation slows heart rate and breathing, reduces metabolism, lowers blood pressure, and even generates the type of brain waves associated with feeling peaceful and calm.

This state of deep relaxation counters the fight-or-flight response. When we are stressed, our heart rate and blood pressure increase dramatically, and adrenaline and other hormones surge through the body. This readies the body to either fight or flee in a situation where our survival depends on one response or the other. Though in the modern world most of us don't face truly life-threatening situations, even minor threats will trigger that same hormonal rush. What's more, even thinking about or recalling a stressful or threatening event can trigger the same chemical cascade. Over time all those chemicals and hormones build up, contributing to what may feel, physically, like a never-ending cycle of stress reactions.

Fortunately, the relaxation response is the physiological antithesis of the fight-or-flight response. This innate response decreases metabolism, heart rate, blood pressure, breathing rate, and muscle tension. You'll learn more about the relaxation response, and how to elicit it, in Chapter 3.

The findings about meditation and the relaxation response were just the first in a series of exciting insights into how the mind affects the body and vice versa. And while the field of mind/body medicine has evolved significantly in the last forty years, its basic premise remains straightforward: Maintaining good health requires that you attend to your mind as well as your body. Negative thoughts and moods can affect you physically, just as pain, stiff joints, and muscles can affect you emotionally. Quiet the mind, and you can calm the body; quiet the body, and you can calm the mind.

According to this philosophy, your health depends on the interplay of a number of factors. Maintaining your heart health means you have to consider blood pressure, cholesterol levels, and family history. But diet, physical activity, stress levels, and social interactions are also important.

■ Assess Your Own Mind/Body Health

You will get the most out of this book if you make the information and advice relevant to your own situation. To do that, be sure to take the quizzes and self-assessment exercises we've included throughout.

A great way to get started is to determine where you are now in terms of your own mind/body health. Try doing the following four exercises. We're hoping that they will not only help you to learn something new about yourself, but will also motivate you to change behaviors that are putting your health—physical, mental, and spiritual—at risk.

Save your initial exercises, because at the end of the book we'll ask that you do them again. You may be pleasantly surprised at how your responses have changed! (To see how some of our patients changed after completing the Cardiac Wellness Program, see the "before" self-portraits on page 10 and "after" self-portraits on page 260. You may want to return to these exercises occasionally to keep yourself on track while trying to make changes in your life.

■ Exercise 1: Draw a Self-Portrait

On a blank piece of paper, draw a picture of yourself. If you have heart disease or some other health condition, depict that in your picture—as well as any treatments you are receiving. Then explain your drawing in a few sentences. (The object of this exercise is not to see whether you are artistic. You can draw a stick figure. It's the process that is most important.) We've included some sample "before" drawings below based on those made by our patients before starting our Cardiac Wellness Program. (For the corresponding "after" drawings, see page 260 in Chapter 9.)

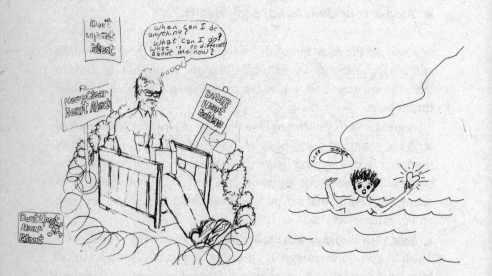

Figures 1 & 2: Two sample "before" self-portraits

■ Exercise 2: Complete the Balance Exercise

Another tool we use in the Cardiac Wellness Program is based on the "Ten Loves" exercise developed by Dr. Sidney B. Simon, a leader in helping people to identify what they value and whether they need more balance in their lifestyles. In this exercise, list the five things that are most important, valuable, and meaningful to you. They can be personal, professional, or spiritual. Then ask yourself the following questions about each of these things:

- When did I do it last?
- Does my illness (or other demands on my time) interfere with my doing it?
- On a scale of 1 to 5 (with 5 being most important), how important is it to me?

			TABLE 1
Things that are important to me:	When did I do it last?	Does my illness/ stress interfere?	How important is it? (Rate from 1 to 5)
1 _____	_____	_____	_____
2 _____	_____	_____	_____
3 _____	_____	_____	_____
4 _____	_____	_____	_____
5 _____	_____	_____	_____

■ Exercise 3: Draw Your Time Pie

Now think about a typical day in your life. Draw a circle on a piece of paper and think of it as representing a twenty-four-hour day. Divide it into "pie" slices to represent how you typically spend your day. Label each slice with the activity and the number of hours or minutes you spend on it. We've included a sample time pie as an example. Obviously, your time pie may vary from one day to the next (weekdays may not resemble weekends, for example). Your particular time pie may also look different if you work nontraditional shifts, such as twelve-hour days.

Take a look at your pie. Is this the way you want to be spending a typical day? Are you spending enough time on the things you value and enjoy? Now draw your ideal time pie. How would your day look if you were living a more balanced life?

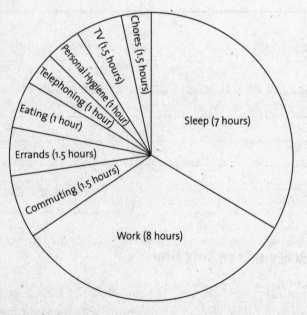

Chores (1.5 hours)

TV (1.5 hours)

Personal Hygiene (1 hour)

Telephoning (1 hour)

Eating (1 hour)

Errands (1.5 hours)

Commuting (1.5 hours)

Sleep (7 hours)

Work (8 hours)

Figure 3: Sample time pie

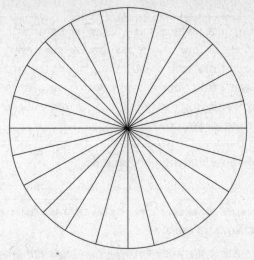

Figure 4: Draw your own time pie

■ Exercise 4: Establish Your Health Contract

Now think about some of the changes you'd like to make so that you can live a more heart-healthy life. In the Cardiac Wellness Program, we ask our patients to sign a health contract. The physical act of writing down specific goals somehow makes them seem more real—and helps ensure that you will actually attain them. Use the following form to help you determine your own personal goals (and then revisit this form occasionally to see if you are making progress). Feel free to revise and personalize it so that you can focus on goals that are important to you.

GOAL 1: LEARN HOW TO BETTER MANAGE STRESS AND EMOTIONS IN DAILY LIFE.

Read Chapters 3, 4, and 5 to help you with this section.
- Practice a relaxation response technique.
  Method: _____

Frequency: _____ Duration: _____
Find a quiet place where you will not be disturbed.

- Practice three to four minirelaxation exercises every day.
- Try to spend time each day thinking about the small things in life that can bring you pleasure: watching a sunset, taking a warm bath, enjoying a candlelit dinner or a walk with a friend. Identify some of your own: _____
- Focus on the areas in your life that *are* going well as much as you do on those that are not going well.

GOAL 2: DEVELOP AN EXERCISE PROGRAM THAT IS COMFORTABLE, CHALLENGING, AND ENJOYABLE.

Read Chapter 8 for more information when filling out this section.
Type: _____
Include both aerobic and strength-training exercises.
Frequency: _____ Duration: _____
Intensity (measured in heart rate or perceived exertion): _____

- Remember to warm up and cool down for five to ten minutes every time you exercise. These are good times to incorporate the yoga stretches we've included.
- Try to accumulate thirty minutes of brisk physical activity on all or most days of the week. (This includes walking to work and walking for enjoyment, as well as housework, yard work, and regular exercise.)

GOAL 3: DEVELOP A HEART-HEALTHY NUTRITION PLAN.

Read Chapters 2, 6, and 7 for more information.
My starting weight is: _____
My short-term weight goal is: _____
My long-term weight goal is: _____
My latest lipid profile is:

Date: _____ TC*: _____ LDL: _____ HDL: _____ Trigs*: _____
Ideal lipids are TC less than 200, LDL less than 130 (no heart disease) or less than 100 (with heart disease or diabetes), HDL greater than 40, Trigs less than 150.

My fat-gram goal is 25 to 35 percent of calories a day, and I will try to consume more monounsaturated and omega-3 fats, and less saturated and trans fats.

My sodium goal is a maximum of 2,000 mg a day.

To reach these goals I will:
  1. Balance my plate.
  2. Eat at least five servings of fruits and vegetables a day.
  3. _____
  4. _____
  5. _____

Sample meal plan for the day:

Breakfast
Whole-grain cereal with skim milk and fruit
Coffee or tea

Lunch
Tossed green salad with avocado and several strips of chicken
Oil (unsaturated) and vinegar dressing
Whole wheat roll
Low-calorie beverage

Healthy snack
Cottage by the Cheese (see recipe, page 275)

Dinner
Grilled salmon
Steamed vegetable medley (broccoli, carrots, snow peas, tomatoes)

---

* TC = total cholesterol count; Trigs = triglycerides

Brown rice
Low-calorie beverage

■ One Step at a Time

Mark Twain once wrote, "Habit is habit, and not to be flung out the window by any man, but coaxed downstairs a step at a time."

Twain had it right. People often talk about "life-changing events," but though certain events may in fact be singular, happening at a particular time and place, change happens over time and takes practice and persistence. Change is also dynamic rather than static. It involves reflecting about your own particular circumstances and beliefs, learning about alternatives, making choices, developing skills, and then making readjustments along the way.

Making changes in behavior is possible no matter what your age, but we're not saying it will be easy. Let's face it, life in the twenty-first century is fast, furious, and frantic. Traffic is stalled, horns blare, E-mail waits, phones ring, deadlines loom. All these external demands and pressures can result in excess stress that worsens symptoms of your heart disease or prevents you from adopting heart-healthy behaviors. That's why we'll suggest real-world strategies that have worked for other people and that may also help you.

The main thing to remember is that change is a process that has to be attended to constantly. The first step, of course, is to identify barriers to change that may be negatively affecting your health, such as a perceived lack of time. The next step, or series of steps, involves setting realistic goals. And the third step is to choose strategies to move toward those goals. As you follow these strategies and adopt new behaviors, you will find the process becomes easier and feels more natural—much like learning to ride a bike.

There is no "one size fits all" to change. You are unique, and you will have to discover the techniques that work for you. A key to our program is cognitive restructuring. The word *cognitive* refers to what you perceive and know about the world; cognitive therapy is based on the premise that much of what we find distressing originates in how we perceive or interpret an event, rather than in the event itself. And many times, our perceptions are negative, unrealistic, and distorted. We hope to help you perceive stress in a new, positive, and manageable way.

Chapter 2

Risky Business

E VERY THIRTY-THREE SECONDS, someone in this country dies from heart disease. It doesn't have to be that way. The factors that contribute to heart disease develop slowly over time. That means you can take immediate steps to improve your health—whether you already have heart disease or are at risk of developing it. But first you have to understand what heart disease is and what factors put you at risk.

Much of the knowledge we have regarding cardiac risk factors comes from the Framingham Heart Study, which has probably done more than any other investigation to change the way we think about heart disease. In 1948, when the Framingham Heart Study began, physicians actually believed that blood pressure *should* increase as people grew older; the theory was that the heart had to work harder over time because people's arteries narrowed with age. The buildup of fatty deposits in the walls of arteries, known medically as atherosclerosis, was thought to be an unavoidable result of growing older. That view changed completely as epidemiologists began to track the health of 5,209 people from Framingham, Massachusetts, a suburb of Boston. Participants in the study ranged in age from thirty to sixty-two, and included both men and women. (The Framingham Heart Study was one of the first heart studies to include women.) Every two years, participants underwent a physical examination, submitted to blood and laboratory tests, and answered questions about their medical history and their habits in lifestyle, diet, and exercise. In later years, two additional studies were started: one that enrolled children of the original participants and another involving minorities.

The Framingham Heart Study and other large-scale epidemiological studies have provided a wealth of scientific evidence that not only biological factors such as high cholesterol and blood pressure put people at risk of developing heart disease; certain lifestyle factors, such as smoking, inactivity, and obesity, also contribute to its development. Newer evidence indicates that psychosocial factors, such as depression, hostility, anger, and low levels of social support, can increase your risk for heart disease whether or not you have any of the traditional risk factors.

That's why we believe that the best way to cultivate heart health is to work with both your mind and your body. Medications and surgery may at times be necessary, but they can only do so much good—especially if you continue to sit on the couch or at the computer and eat foods high in saturated fats or trans fats, and deal ineffectively with stressful situations.

In this chapter, we'll briefly review both the traditional and newly identified risk factors for heart disease. Some risk factors are more significant than others; some can be changed, while others cannot. Still, everyone can make positive changes to take better control of his or her own heart health. To see why, you first have to understand how heart disease develops in the first place.

■ Anatomy of Heart Attack

The adult heart, or myocardium, is a robust muscle about the size of your clenched fist and tucked behind the breastbone. It con-

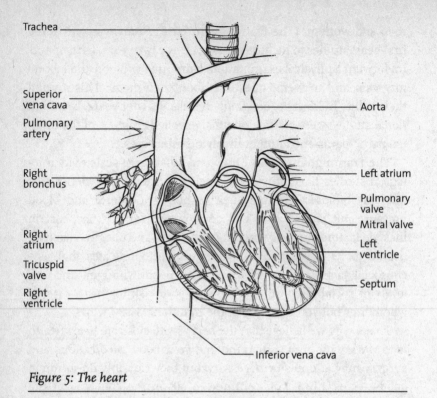

Trachea

Superior vena cava

Pulmonary artery

Right bronchus

Right atrium

Tricuspid valve

Right ventricle

Aorta

Left atrium

Pulmonary valve

Mitral valve

Left ventricle

Septum

Inferior vena cava

Figure 5: The heart

tains four internal chambers: two upper chambers called atria, which act as reservoirs to collect blood, and two lower chambers called ventricles, which pump blood out to the lungs and to the rest of the body. As seen in Figure 5, oxygen-depleted blood travels through the inferior and superior vena cava to the right atrium and then flows down into the right ventricle. Thereafter it is pumped through the pulmonary artery to the lungs for reoxygenation. Meanwhile freshly oxygenated blood travels via the pulmonary veins to the left side of your heart. This oxygen-rich blood flows first into the left atrium and then into the left ventricle, where it is finally pumped out the aorta to flow throughout the body.

Like all muscles, the heart requires a constant supply of blood

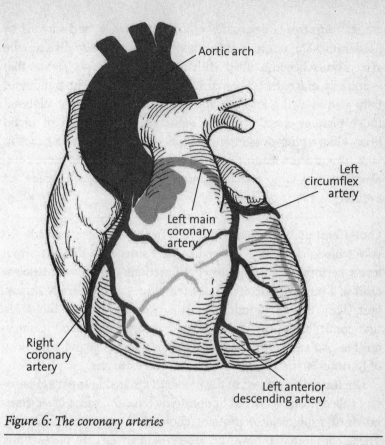

Figure 6: The coronary arteries

and oxygen in order to stay healthy so that it can do its job properly. And in spite of its overwhelming importance in the body, the heart has only two major arteries, the right coronary artery and the left main coronary artery, which quickly branches into two smaller arteries (the left circumflex artery and the left anterior descending artery). Like the branch of a tree, each major artery divides into progressively smaller arteries that carry blood to the heart-muscle cells.

Heart disease begins with a blockage in one or more of the coronary arteries. This process is known as *atherosclerosis,* which comes from two Greek words *athere,* or porridge, and *sclerosis,* or hardening. The name is accurate; in coronary artery disease, the artery walls become filled with deposits known as *plaque* that eventually make the artery hard, stiff, and narrow. The buildup of fatty plaque in the arteries, and the formation of blood clots on those plaques, results in the reduction or cessation of blood flow—like a plug clogging up a pipe—and this causes a heart attack. The process leading to a heart attack, however, is more complex than this simple analogy suggests, involving a "cascade" of events.

Cholesterol buildup: The first event in the coronary cascade involves blood cholesterol, a waxlike fatty substance that at normal levels performs a number of vital functions in the body. Cholesterol is a building block of cell membranes, the critically important "skin" that surrounds cells. It is used to make the bile acids that contribute to the digestion and absorption of food. Cholesterol is also an important precursor for vitamin D and a number of hormones, including testosterone and estrogen.

Cholesterol is carried in the bloodstream inside spherical particles called *lipoproteins.* All lipoproteins have the same basic components: triglycerides, protein, cholesterol, and phospholipids. These components, however, are present in varying proportions depending on the type of lipoprotein. Two lipoproteins in particular are relevant to heart disease: low-density lipoproteins (LDLs), sometimes referred to as "bad" cholesterol, and high-density lipoproteins (HDLs), also known as "good" cholesterol. (For ideal lipoprotein levels, see Table 2 on page 30.)

About two-thirds of blood cholesterol comes in the form of LDL, which contains more fat than protein. The higher the level of LDL cholesterol, the greater the risk for coronary artery disease, since excess LDL cholesterol lodges in the artery walls. It may be helpful to imagine LDL as a full dump truck spilling fat and cholesterol as it travels through the bloodstream.

HDL, which contains more protein than fat, protects the heart by carrying cholesterol away from the arteries to the liver, where it is metabolized into bile salts that exit the body harmlessly through the intestinal tract. To return to the analogy used earlier, HDL is like an empty dump truck that picks up the fat and cholesterol left behind by LDL cholesterol and delivers it to the liver so that it can be excreted from the body. Anything that increases your level of HDL cholesterol will help you reduce your risk for heart disease.

Plaques develop: A plaque is an accumulation of fat, cholesterol, and inflammatory cells inside an artery wall. Until a few years ago, physicians thought that atherosclerotic plaques were passive plugs that block arteries mechanically—and the bigger the plug, the worse for your heart. But recent research has revealed just the opposite: Although smaller plaques may only narrow coronary arteries by 40 to 60 percent, they are actually more dangerous than larger plaques that narrow them by 70 to 80 percent. Smaller plaques are covered with thin, fibrous caps that are more vulnerable and can easily rupture, while larger ones tend to be covered with tough caps made of collagen (a connective tissue). *We now know that two-thirds of all heart attacks result from the smaller, more vulnerable plaques.*

Plaques begin to form when the inner lining of the arterial wall, or endothelium, is injured, accelerating the passage of LDL cholesterol out of the blood and into the artery wall. Further injury occurs when LDL itself is damaged by free radicals, highly reactive molecules that make LDL more volatile. (For more information on free radicals, see page 156.) The damaged endothelial cells send out distress signals that summon immune system cells known as macrophages and monocytes to the scene. These white blood cells ingest the LDL and, in the process, become enlarged, fat-laden foam cells that form the plaques of atherosclerosis and provoke still further inflammation in the coronary artery.

It is not clear what causes a plaque to rupture, but it appears

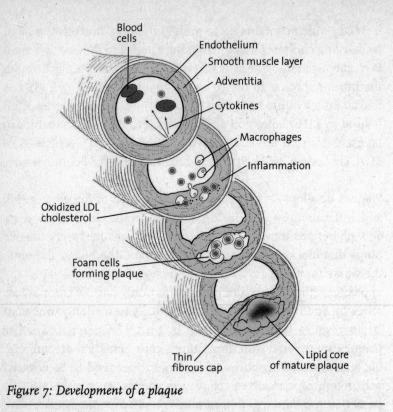

Blood
cells

Endothelium

Smooth muscle layer

Adventitia

Cytokines

Macrophages

Inflammation

Oxidized LDL
cholesterol

Foam cells
forming plaque

Thin
fibrous cap

Lipid core
of mature plaque

Figure 7: Development of a plaque

that any one of a number of physical and emotional triggers can initiate the process. Once the process begins, immune system T cells, which normally defend the body, instead issue commands that end up harming it. Activated T cells secrete gamma interferon, a molecule that simultaneously signals smooth muscle cells in the blood vessel wall to stop producing new collagen while also ordering macrophages to produce enzymes that dissolve existing collagen. As a result the cap covering the plaque degrades and the plaque ruptures.

Clot formation and heart attack: Once a plaque ruptures, additional immune system cells rush to the scene, setting off the final

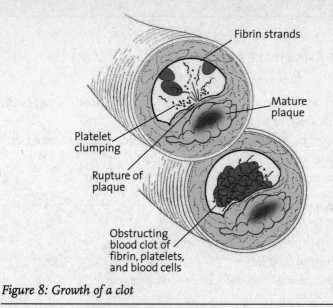

Figure 8: Growth of a clot

events that lead to a heart attack. First, inflammatory cells send a signal that attracts platelets, the fragmentary blood cells that initiate the clotting process. Once on the scene, platelets clump together and adhere to the surface of the ruptured plaque, triggering the interaction of blood proteins, such as fibrin, which serve as clotting factors. A clot, or thrombus, made up of clotting factors, platelets, and red blood cells, then forms.

When a clot blocks an artery completely, the result is a heart attack, known medically as a *myocardial infarction* (death of heart tissue). Although symptoms vary, they are usually intense and generally last fifteen minutes or longer. Some men report severe chest pain, likening it to an elephant sitting on their chest; others feel as though they have pulled a muscle in their chest or arm. (Women commonly report different symptoms, such as gastrointestinal distress, an ache between the breasts, or shortness of breath.) Familiarize yourself with the symptoms of a heart attack for both sexes listed in Sidebar 3, page 26. If you ever think you

---

SIDEBAR 3

SYMPTOMS OF A HEART ATTACK

In Men:
- Pain or discomfort that radiates to shoulders or arms, upper back (scapula area), or to neck and jaw
- Uncomfortable pressure, tightness, fullness, or ache at center of the chest
- Shortness of breath, sweating, nausea, or dizziness

In Women:
- Pain in both arms or shoulders
- Chest cramping, dull pain between breasts
- Shortness of breath
- Gastric burning/pain or feeling of indigestion
- Lower abdominal pain
- Severe fatigue, tiredness, or depression

---

are having a heart attack, call your local emergency response number (usually 911) and ask to be taken to the hospital immediately. Do not drive yourself!

Additional heart problems: Atherosclerosis and the resulting interruption of blood flow, known medically as *ischemia,* can adversely affect the heart in other ways. The chest pain known as *angina* is one of the most common heart problems, affecting more than 6 million Americans. People may experience angina when fatty deposits of cholesterol and plaque significantly narrow the artery but still allow blood to flow through. As a result, far less oxygen-rich blood gets through the artery. Angina is usually triggered by exercise or emotional stress, when the body's demand for oxygen increases and the heart works harder. Symptoms resemble those of a heart attack and include sensations of discomfort, pressure, squeezing, burning, fullness, heaviness, tightness, and aching—even indigestion. The pain may be centered in the chest or radiate outward to the throat, jaws, shoulders, or arms. These symptoms generally last only a few minutes and are usually alleviated if you rest (which reduces the heart's demand for oxygen) or take sublingual nitroglycerin (which improves blood flow). The heart muscle sustains no actual damage in angina, and if you experience this chest pain it does not necessarily mean you will suffer a heart attack. Even so, take it as a warning sign that you may be at risk for a coronary event. Many of our patients participate in the Cardiac Wellness Program after experiencing angina, heeding it as a wake-up call about overall heart health.

■ Know Your Risk Factors

As frightening as it may be to read about, the development of heart disease is predictable—and largely preventable. The first step is to identify the factors that put you at risk for heart disease, and then take steps to reduce your risk.

SIDEBAR 4

RISK FACTORS FOR HEART DISEASE

Factors that cannot be changed:
Age
Gender
Family history of heart disease

Physical factors that can be changed:
Exposure to tobacco smoke
High blood pressure
Elevated blood cholesterol levels
Inactivity
Diabetes
Obesity

Psychological factors that can be changed:
Anger and hostility
Depression
Social support

Factors that are still under investigation:
Fibrinogen
Homocysteine
Inflammatory agents
  C-reactive protein
  Chlamydia pneumoniae

Of course, you have no control over some factors, such as your age or a family history of heart disease. But you can control other factors, at least to some degree. And while there are no guarantees, reducing your risk factors does improve your chance of avoiding heart disease.

■ The Major Traditional Risk Factors

Cigarette smoking: If you smoke cigarettes, you double your risk of heart disease—making this the single most preventable risk factor for cardiac disease. Other tobacco products, such as pipe tobacco and cigars, and exposure to secondhand smoke may also increase your risk for heart disease (and cancer). Smoking harms the heart in three ways. It promotes atherosclerosis, possibly by damaging the artery walls so that cholesterol deposits accumulate more easily. It also reduces the level of HDL cholesterol and encourages blood clots to form. Fortunately, smokers who quit reduce their risk for heart disease almost immediately. Recent research shows that your risk will decrease by 50 percent one year after quitting.

TIPS TO HELP QUIT SMOKING

Here are some tips based on material from the American Lung Association.

- Make a list of the health hazards and other disadvantages of smoking.
- Make a list of the benefits of quitting. Be specific.
- Pick a quit date and stick to it. Throw out all cigarettes, ashtrays, matchbooks, and lighters.
- Get other smokers in your household or workplace to join you in quitting.
- Avoid high-risk situations like cocktail parties or stressful social or work-related encounters until you are secure in your success.
- Find other ways to relieve tension, such as exercise, meditation, deep breathing, prayer, or social support.
- Take one day at a time.
- If you don't succeed on your first try, try again. It usually takes people two to three attempts to quit smoking completely.
- Talk with your doctor about nicotine replacement (the patch or gum) or bupropion HCl (brand names: Wellbutrin SR, Zyban).
- When you get the urge to smoke, remind yourself that it will pass whether you smoke or not. You just need to get through the urge.
- Keep low-calorie snacks in the house.

Cholesterol: As total cholesterol levels increase, so does the risk for heart attack. People with cholesterol levels of 240 mg/dL or higher, for instance, are twice as likely to have a heart attack as are those with a cholesterol level of 200 mg/dL. For every 1 percent reduction you achieve in your total cholesterol, you reduce your risk for heart disease by 2 percent—so this is a wise health investment. But since not all cholesterol is alike (see page 22), you have to act strategically by taking measures to increase levels of "good" HDL while decreasing "bad" LDL. Also try to lower your levels of triglycerides, the major form in which fat is stored in food and in the body's tissue, because high levels increase your risk for heart disease. For specific cholesterol recommendations, see Table 2 below.

High blood pressure: One in three American adults already has high blood pressure, and Framingham Heart Study researchers recently warned that nine out of ten people older than fifty-five are at risk of developing it. That is worrisome, because people with high blood pressure are more than twice as likely to suffer a heart

TABLE 2

IDEAL CHOLESTEROL AND BLOOD PRESSURE LEVELS

	Ideal Levels	Ways to Improve Toward Ideal
Total cholesterol	<200 mg/dL	Diet low in saturated fat, trans fat, and cholesterol

LDL
   Person without
   heart disease
	<130 mg/dL	Diet low in saturated fat, trans fat, and cholesterol

Person with heart
   disease and/or
   diabetes
	<100 mg/dL	Diet low in saturated fat, trans fat, and cholesterol

HDL	>40 mg/dL	Exercise, weight loss, and smoking cessation
Triglycerides	<150 mg/dL	Diet low in total fat, carbohydrates, and alcohol
Blood pressure	≤120/80 mm Hg	Weight loss, smoking cessation, reduction of stress, increase in physical activity, lower alcohol intake, lower salt intake, and eat more fruits and vegetables

attack as those with normal blood pressure. Recently, the National Heart, Lung, and Blood Institute issued new guidelines for blood pressure. A new category, Prehypertension (120–139/80–89 mm Hg), has been added. Fortunately, just a 1 mm Hg decline in diastolic blood pressure can reduce a person's risk for heart disease by 2 to 3 percent.

Your blood pressure reading has two parts, systolic blood pressure (the top number) and diastolic blood pressure (the bottom number). The systolic number represents the pressure while the heart is beating, and the diastolic number represents the pressure while the heart is refilling with blood between beats. There is no single "normal" blood pressure reading; instead, blood pressure readings range from optimal to high, with average blood pressure of 120/80 mm Hg. In general, the lower your blood pressure, the better.

Inactivity: Sedentary lifestyle almost doubles a person's risk for heart disease, which means that lack of exercise is nearly as dangerous to the heart as smoking, abnormal cholesterol levels, or hypertension. Fortunately, recent research has shown that even moderate exercise can substantially reduce the incidence of cardiac events. Try to accumulate at least thirty minutes of moderate activity a day on most days of the week. (For much more on exercise, see Chapter 8.)

■ Additional Risk Factors

Age: About four of every five people who die from heart attacks are older than age sixty-five. The risk for heart attack begins to increase for men after age forty-five and for women after fifty-five.

Gender: Heart disease is the leading cause of death in both men and women in the United States. Before age sixty, one in five

American men—but only one in seventeen women—has had a cardiac event. Beyond age sixty, as many women die of heart disease as men. In part, this statistical convergence is due to women's lower levels of heart-protecting estrogen as they enter menopause, but it also reflects social changes that have increased women's exposure to risk factors such as smoking, physical inactivity, and mental stress.

Family history: Heart disease tends to run in families, but this risk is often blown out of proportion. When disregarding lifestyle factors such as smoking, diet, and inactivity, investigators for the Framingham Heart Study estimate that having a family history of heart disease increases an individual's risk by about 25 percent. To put this in perspective, a family history of heart disease is only about one-tenth as dangerous as smoking cigarettes. Moreover it takes a strong history (a father or brother afflicted before age fifty-five or a mother or sister before age sixty-five) to increase a person's risk.

Diabetes: Nine out of ten people who are diabetic have Type 2 diabetes (also known as "adult onset" diabetes), which develops as people gain weight and become resistant to the effects of insulin, a hormone that helps metabolize blood sugar. (Insulin dependent diabetes, the other form of the disease, involves a deficiency in insulin production, not a resistance to its effects.) Either form is risky to the heart: Two-thirds of people who have diabetes die of some form of heart or blood vessel disease.

It is not completely understood how diabetes contributes to heart disease, but it is probably through a combination of effects. For example, over time diabetes lowers "good" HDL cholesterol, increases triglyceride levels, and slightly increases "bad" LDL cholesterol. Elevated blood sugar levels also cause glycation—the attachment of glucose to proteins and lipids—and an increased tendency for oxidation, which promotes atherosclerosis. Diabetes may also damage nerves in the heart, so that a person may not feel pain or discomfort from angina or a heart attack.

Fortunately, the most common form of the disease, non-insulin dependent diabetes, can be controlled (or even prevented) by diet, weight loss, regular aerobic exercise, and stress management. If you have diabetes, work with your doctor to keep your blood sugar levels as close to normal as possible. The goal is to achieve a "fasting" glucose reading of 80 to 126 mg/dL (determined by a blood test taken after an overnight fast of at least eight hours) or a glycosylated hemoglobin (AIC) of between 4.8 percent and 6 percent. (The glycosylated hemoglobin test assesses average blood sugar levels over the preceding two to three months by measuring the amount of glucose that adheres to hemoglobin.)

Obesity: Maintaining a healthy body weight can reduce your risk for heart disease by at least one-third and possibly one-half. All

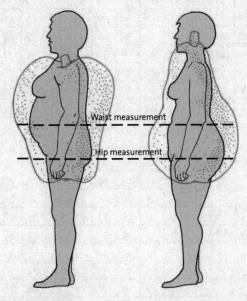

Figure 9: Apples and pears

forms of obesity are bad for health, but excessive upper body fat (the "apple" shape) is more dangerous to the heart than lower body obesity (the "pear" shape). That's why losing inches from your waist may be more important than dropping pounds on the scale.

You can use two simple tests to determine your body-weight composition. First, to determine your waist-to-hip ratio (WHR):

1. With your abdomen relaxed, measure your waist in inches at its narrowest (usually around the navel).
2. Measure your hips in inches at the widest point (usually around the largest part of your buttocks).
3. Divide the waist measurement by the hip measurement to determine your WHR.

WEIGHT

HEIGHT	100	110	120	130	140	150	160	170	180	190	200	210	220	230	240	250
5'0"	20	21	23	25	27	29	31	33	35	37	39	41	43	45	47	49
5'1"	19	21	23	25	26	28	30	32	34	36	38	40	42	43	45	47
5'2"	18	20	22	24	26	27	29	31	33	35	37	38	40	42	44	46
5'3"	18	19	21	23	25	27	28	30	32	34	35	37	39	41	43	44
5'4"	17	19	21	22	24	26	27	29	31	33	34	36	38	39	41	43
5'5"	17	18	20	22	23	25	27	28	30	32	33	35	37	38	40	42
5'6"	16	18	19	21	23	24	26	27	29	31	32	34	36	37	39	40
5'7"	16	17	19	20	22	23	25	27	28	30	31	33	34	36	38	39
5'8"	15	17	18	20	21	23	24	26	27	29	30	32	33	35	36	38
5'9"	15	16	18	19	21	22	24	25	27	28	30	31	32	34	35	37
5'10"	14	16	17	19	20	22	23	24	26	27	29	30	32	33	34	36
5'11"	14	15	17	18	20	21	22	24	25	26	27	28	30	32	33	35
6'0"	14	15	16	18	19	20	22	23	24	26	27	28	30	31	33	34
6'1"	13	15	16	17	18	20	21	22	24	25	26	28	29	30	32	33
6'2"	13	14	15	17	18	19	21	22	23	24	26	27	28	30	31	32
6'3"	12	14	15	16	17	19	20	21	22	24	25	26	27	29	30	31
6'4"	12	13	15	16	17	18	19	21	22	23	24	26	27	28	29	30

Figure 10: Body mass index (BMI)

The risk for heart attack and stroke increases substantially in women with ratios above 0.85 and in men with ratios above 0.95. For example, men with ratios above 1.0 have twice the death rate of men with ratios below 0.85.

The second method, body mass index (BMI), takes both your height and weight into consideration. Although there is a formula for calculating BMI, an easier method may be to consult the chart in Figure 10, page 34. To find your BMI, first identify your weight (to the nearest ten pounds) in the top row of the chart. Next, move your finger down the column below that weight until you come to the row that corresponds to your height. The number at the intersection of your height and weight is your BMI. You should aim for a BMI of between 18.5 and 24, the range that is considered normal. A BMI between 25 and 29 is considered overweight, and a value of 30 or more is defined as obese.

Elevated homocysteine: In 1992, the Physicians' Health Study reported that elevated levels of homocysteine, an amino acid that is a by-product of methionine (a protein found in food), tripled the risk for heart attack, even after other risk factors had been taken into account. Additional studies have added to researchers' concerns. It appears that high levels of homocysteine may harm arteries by damaging endothelial cells in the inner layer of the artery wall or by stimulating abnormal growth of smooth muscle cells in the middle layer of the artery wall. Homocysteine may also activate the blood clotting system, thereby promoting the formation of clots that are ultimately responsible for most heart attacks. Ideally, homocysteine levels should be under 9 to 10 micromol per liter, measured through a blood test.

Many studies reveal that people with high homocysteine levels are deficient in the B vitamins: folic acid, B_6, and B_{12}. Having a balanced diet that includes at least five servings of fruits and vegetables a day, or taking multivitamin or B-complex supplements, can reduce homocysteine levels to normal. There already is some direct evidence that increasing intake of these B vitamins, either through diet or vitamin supplements, can reduce the progression of atherosclerosis. The Swiss Heart Study (a randomized controlled trial) demonstrated that patients undergoing angioplasty who received a combination of folic acid, B_{12}, and B_6 (a combination commonly used to treat high homocysteine levels) required fewer future angioplasty procedures. For tips on how to maintain a well-balanced diet, see Chapters 6 and 7.

Inflammatory damage: Inflammation is the body's protective response to injury, infection, or allergy. But when inflammation occurs in coronary arteries—in response to damage inflicted by oxidized LDL cholesterol—it can set the stage for atherosclerosis. Although researchers are still trying to determine all the mechanisms of inflammatory damage, a few clear suspects have emerged.

One potential culprit is C-reactive protein, a by-product of inflammation. In a 1997 report in the *New England Journal of Medicine,* men with the highest C-reactive protein levels were nearly three times more likely to have a heart attack than men with the lowest levels. The following year, the Harvard Women's Health Study found that C-reactive protein predicts heart disease risk in women as well. Although the magnitude of risk varies from study to study, people with the highest C-reactive protein levels appear to be three to five times more likely to develop heart disease than people with the lowest levels. To make the situation even more complicated, the standard C-reactive protein test (once used to diagnose rheumatic fever) is not sensitive enough to detect specific levels of the protein that put the heart at risk. Your best bet is to ask your physician about whether you should be tested for C-reactive protein. If you should, ask for the high-sensitivity test, which can detect even subtle changes in C-reactive protein levels. The current research suggests that a level of less than 1 mg/L indicates low cardiovascular risk; 1–3, moderate risk; and above 3, high risk (about twice that of someone with a level below 1).

Another possible contender is *Chlamydia pneumoniae,* a bacterium that can cause pneumonia, bronchitis, and sinus infections. This bacterium routinely shows up in atherosclerotic plaques. But that doesn't necessarily mean the microbes cause the plaques to build up. They might just be innocent bystanders that are attracted to atherosclerotic areas. If *C. pneumoniae* does pan out as an agent of inflammation, scientists may one day add antibiotics to their arsenal of standard treatments for coronary artery disease, although so far the few studies of antibiotics for atherosclerosis have produced disappointing results.

■ Psychosocial Factors

Only half of heart disease cases diagnosed in the United States can be explained by the traditional risk factors we've just discussed. It is not yet clear what triggers a heart attack in people who do not have the traditional risk factors. One theory is that psychosocial factors, such as depression, hostility, anger, and low levels of social support, may have a more significant impact on heart health than previously believed. Each of these negative emotions places stress on the heart, which can raise blood pressure, decrease the heart's pumping ability, trigger abnormal heart rhythms, and activate the blood-clotting system.

Depression: Many people are surprised to learn that depression is not only a risk factor for heart disease but that it can adversely affect prognosis. A number of research studies actually suggest that depression may be the psychological state most likely to harm your heart—giving all new meaning to the term *brokenhearted.*

Everyone gets depressed occasionally. A major life change, such as the loss of a job, or personal grief, such as the death of a loved one, typically causes situational depression. But most people experience mild symptoms, such as reduced energy and feeling blue, for only a temporary period. Gradually, they recover their resilience and their mood improves. A major depressive episode goes well beyond a temporary mood change and actually interferes with your ability to carry out normal daily activities, such as working, eating, and sleeping.

It is clear that depression has an adverse effect on the heart, although researchers are still trying to quantify and better understand the relationship. One in five people recently diagnosed with heart disease is depressed. Studies have shown that depression increases the risk of suffering a heart attack and the likelihood of dying from heart disease.

Why is depression so hard on the heart? Depressed people do not suffer from advanced disease more often than other people, but for some reason they don't recover as well. The underlying mechanisms for this phenomenon are not clear, but we have a number of theories.

One possible reason is behavioral. It may be that depressed people are less likely to take steps to change a risky behavior, such as smoking, or to comply with treatment regimens. Another is biological. A number of studies have shown that depression may decrease heart rate variability and increase the likelihood of life-threatening irregular heartbeats, known as *arrhythmias*. Depression also increases blood platelet aggregation, promoting the formation of clots that can clog arteries. And depression has been associated with dysfunction in the mood hormone serotonin, which encourages platelets to stick together, exacerbating the tendency to form blood clots.

Fortunately, you can take steps to relieve depression—and the first step may be a good, brisk walk. (One group of researchers has found that aerobic exercise is as effective as a certain antidepressant in treating older people with depression, for instance. For more on this study and other beneficial aspects of exercise, see Chapter 8.) It may also help to increase your social support (see Chapter 5). Of course, if symptoms are severe or persist, see your health care provider about medications or counseling that

---

SYMPTOMS OF MAJOR DEPRESSION

Do you have the temporary blues or something more significant in terms of mood change? If you have experienced five or more of the following symptoms nearly every day for at least two weeks and have not endured a significant loss (such as the death of a loved one), you may be suffering from major depression. This may be true especially if there is no medical reason for the symptoms, and if they are impairing your ability to function normally. Ask your doctor for help and/or a referral to a mental health specialist if you have experienced the following symptoms according to the profile above.

- Feeling depressed, sad, or "empty"
- Lack of interest or pleasure in activities, even those formerly enjoyed
- Loss of appetite and weight or ravenous appetite and weight gain
- Inability to sleep or oversleeping
- Feeling restless and agitated or sluggish
- Low energy, fatigue, or burnout
- Feeling guilty or worthless
- Inability to think, concentrate, or make decisions
- Suicidal thoughts or attempts

---

may help. There are many effective treatments for depression, and there is no reason to be in pain—or to put any additional strain on your heart.

Low social support: What about lonely hearts? Health care providers have long recognized that people who have a network of friends and loved ones report having better health than people who don't. In the past twenty years or so, an increasing body of research has indicated that maintaining a strong level of social support can also provide a buffer against heart disease, while lack of human connection can significantly increase risk.

To understand why this is true, think of when you felt most relaxed and happy over the past week. Chances are, the events you remember will involve interaction with one or more people: a night out with your spouse, perhaps, or lunch with a friend. People are social beings. Many of us marry and start families. Others may remain unmarried but enjoy close bonds with friends. We may attend a house of worship regularly or join a sports team, a support group, or a club to pursue a favorite hobby. Yet all too often in modern society, we have to contend with multiple forces that tend to drive us apart: tightly packed schedules, competing demands, and deadlines. The results? Eating at your desk so that you can meet a deadline, rather than meeting a friend for lunch. Less time spent with the family at home. Vacations canceled or interrupted by work demands. Broken marriages, soured relationships.

All of this takes a physical toll on a person. Various studies have concluded that death rates are higher for single people than they are for married people, and that retired men are nearly twice as likely to suffer a fatal heart attack as men who are still working, even after adjusting for age and medical history.

Not all the news is bad. A number of research studies have also examined the beneficial impact of social relations on heart health. The findings may surprise you. A study conducted by researchers at the Honolulu Heart Program asked 4,653 men of Japanese descent about their social interactions with relatives and coworkers, and their membership in religious and social groups. The study found that the larger a man's social network was, the less likely he was to experience angina, a heart attack, or any type of heart disease. Investigators analyzing outcomes for the ten thousand men participating in the Israeli Heart Disease Study concluded that men suffering from high anxiety levels, but who also felt supported and loved by their wives, were less likely to experience angina than men with similar anxiety levels who did not enjoy such spousal support. Other research has shown that people who receive emotional support after a heart attack may recover better than people who do not have such support.

It is not clear why social support promotes heart health, but studies have demonstrated that a lack of such support is associated with particular risk factors for heart disease. One study found that people with the fewest social interactions also had the highest levels of fibrinogen, which enhances blood clotting and thus can increase risk for heart disease. Another found that people who felt they had low social support at work were more likely to have higher systolic blood pressure and heart rates than people who enjoyed higher levels of support. Interestingly, blood pressure and heart rate increased both at work and at home for those who reported low levels of social support.

Friends and family clearly matter when it comes to your heart. If you are feeling isolated, determine where you can connect with people in your community. Join a club or attend a place of worship. Even pets can have an amazingly beneficial effect on your heart. Studies have shown that having a pet or spending time with a friendly animal can lower blood pressure and reduce cardiac reactivity, even in stressful situations.

Anger and hostility: The phrase *type A behavior* was coined in the late 1950s by two California cardiologists, Dr. Meyer Friedman and Dr. Ray Rosenman, although this type of behavior was first described clinically more than a century earlier. Friedman and Rosenman not only coined the term, however, but also found a way to categorize aspects of type A behavior that might contribute to heart disease. The two doctors noticed that people who were hard charging, competitive, impatient, aggressive, and felt pressured for time also tended to have heart disease. But as they and others continued such research, the type A behavior hypothesis was refined. It turns out that not all type A people are alike. Some are quite happy and energized as they charge through life, constantly checking their watches. Others are not.

It now appears that the most toxic elements of type A behavior are subcomponents of the personality profile, such as anger, hostility, and cynical thinking. Research shows that people who regularly display such negative mood states are more likely to develop heart disease and more likely to die from it.

Hostility also exacerbates the heart risk posed by other factors such as depression. Research indicates that people who are hostile as well as depressed are more likely to die after suffering a heart attack. Some estimate that one out of five people in the general population are hostile enough to increase their risk for heart disease. Such hostility manifests itself not only in sour and cynical moods, but also in hyperaggressiveness and explosive speech patterns that ignite frequently and after even minimal provocation.

Anger can also be deadly to the heart. Various studies estimate that anywhere from 4 to 18 percent of heart attacks may be triggered by severe emotional stress that occurs immediately beforehand. A study involving 1,623 people who had recently suffered a heart attack found that 8 percent had experienced intense anger in the twenty-four hours preceding their attack, and an additional 2.4 percent experienced the same feelings in the two hours preceding it. Family arguments, work conflicts, and legal problems lead the list of events that triggered an angry reaction. (For tips on how to deal with emotions, see Chapter 5.)

It is not entirely clear why negative emotional states such as anger and hostility harm the heart, but several studies point to the mind/body connection. Negative mood states have adverse physiological effects on the heart, resulting in increased heart rate, blood pressure, and other harmful changes.

Although we'll be discussing the mind/body connection as it concerns heart disease in much greater detail in Chapter 4, a brief summary is appropriate now. When you feel stress, you activate the fight-or-flight response, during which three physical changes occur. First, you become tense, as muscles in your jaw, shoulders, and back tighten. Second, the autonomic nervous system is activated, unleashing a flood of hormones that affect the functioning of internal organs. Among other responses, you sweat, your blood pressure increases, and your cholesterol and triglyceride levels rise. Third, the psychoneuroendocrine system is activated, unleashing additional hormones that increase blood sugar, promote calcium retention, and put the immune system into overdrive. All the hormones released during the stress response normally perform useful roles in the body, but they can become harmful in excessive amounts or if they circulate for too long.

■ Getting Better

Oddly enough, the very complexity of heart disease is what offers people hope. Just as there are multiple risk factors, so too you can employ numerous strategies to improve the health of your heart. To return to the image of the three-legged stool we introduced in Chapter 1, no single strategy is likely to be sufficient on its own; instead, you'll do best if you employ all three. We'll provide a quick overview here.

■ Medications

A number of different medications are used to prevent or treat heart disease. Some medication regimens can even limit the damage from a heart attack or help prevent a second one. Consult with your doctor about which medications are best for you and how long you should take them. (Generally speaking, many of these medications should be taken for the long term and perhaps for the rest of your life.) Remember to ask about cost and side effects, since this information may factor into your decision making.

Cholesterol-lowering medications: In an ideal world, lifestyle changes would always be rewarded by excellent blood cholesterol levels; in reality, it's not necessarily so. Some people find that despite improvements in diet and exercise, their cholesterol level remains high. If this is true in your case, discuss the pros and cons of cholesterol-lowering medications with your doctor.

Statins: These medications work by inhibiting a liver enzyme that is responsible for producing cholesterol. When the enzyme is inhibited, less cholesterol is produced; to compensate, the liver takes up extra LDL cholesterol from the blood. As a result, both total cholesterol and harmful LDL cholesterol levels fall. Some of the statins also lower triglycerides, which have been implicated in heart disease. Members of this drug family include lovastatin (Mevacor), pravastatin (Pravachol), simvastatin (Zocor), fluvastatin (Lescol), and atorvastatin (Lipitor). Recent studies show that statins may also make plaque more stable and less vulnerable.

Fibrates: The fibrates, or fibric acid derivatives, are medications that lower cholesterol by reducing its synthesis in the body. Fibrates include gemfibrozil (Lopid) and fenofibrate (Tricor) and are particularly useful for patients with high blood triglyceride levels.

Bile acid–binding resins: These are the oldest cholesterol-lowering drugs, and they include cholestyramine (Questran, Questran Light) and colestipol (Colestid). These medications act by sequestering bile acids in the intestines and preventing them from entering the blood and traveling to the liver, where they would ordinarily be converted into cholesterol.

Niacin: A form of this B vitamin, known as nicotinic acid, is useful in lowering trigylceride levels and LDL cholesterol while increasing levels of HDL cholesterol. (In fact, nicotinic acid raises HDL more than any other cholesterol-lowering medication. It is also relatively low in cost.) Sample brand names include Endur-Acin, Niacor, and Nicolar. Don't try to self-medicate by increasing your intake of vitamin supplements, however, because the form of niacin they contain can, at high doses, harm your liver.

Cardiovascular medications: Many drugs are used to treat people already diagnosed with cardiovascular disease. When used appropriately, these drugs can decrease symptoms and improve cardiac function, but only a few can help prevent heart attacks.

Aspirin: Aspirin inhibits blood clot formation. For patients who have already had angina or a heart attack, aspirin reduces the risk for future heart attacks by about 25 percent. But aspirin's role in reducing the risk for a first heart attack in people without known heart disease is less clear. Studies suggest that aspirin does not reduce the formation of new atherosclerotic plaques but that it does prevent clots from blocking arteries already partially narrowed by old plaque.

ACE inhibitors: Over the last ten years, angiotensin-converting enzyme (ACE) inhibitors have been widely prescribed for high blood pressure and are now standard care for people with heart failure. These drugs prevent angiotensin, a blood vessel–constricting protein, from forming. ACE inhibitors thus lower blood pressure by helping blood vessels relax and dilate. Recent research indicates ACE inhibitors may also prevent the development of diabetes in some people and reduce the risk for heart attack and stroke. Members of this drug family include captopril (Capoten), enalapril (Vasotec), lisinopril (Zestril, Prinivil), ramipril (Altace), and many others.

Angiotensin receptor blockers: These cousins of ACE inhibitors work in a slightly different way to restore normal blood flow, by preventing angiotensin from exerting its blood vessel–constricting effects in the body. If you have developed significant side effects while taking an ACE inhibitor (typically, a persistent cough), your physician may prescribe an angiotensin receptor blocker (ARB) instead. ARBs include candesartan (Atacand), irbesartan (Avapro), losartan (Cozaar), and valsartan (Diovan).

Beta-blockers: These medications have an important role in preventing another heart attack in people who have already had one. As a class, beta-blockers take their name from the effect they have of blocking the action of norepinephrine, or adrenaline, which is a beta-adrenergic substance. They are often used to reduce blood pressure or slow heart rate. Doctors can choose from among more than ten different varieties, determining the dose and frequency of therapy best suited to each patient. Beta-blockers include atenolol (Tenormin), labetalol (Normodyne), metoprolol (Lopressor), propranolol (Inderal), and sotalol (Betapace).

Calcium channel blockers: These medications interfere with the absorption of calcium in the heart muscle and blood vessels, causing muscle walls to relax and dilate. As a result, the heartbeat slows and blood pressure falls. Drugs in this class include diltiazem (Cardizem, Dilacor-XR), nifedipine (Adalat, Procardia), and verapamil (Calan, Isoptin, Verelan).

Nitrate medications: Probably the best-known medication in this class is nitroglycerin, although there are others such as isosorbide dinitrate (Isordil). Nitrate medications work as vasodilators, which widen the coronary arteries and improve blood flow.

Thrombolytic therapy: Medications that dissolve blood clots are known medically as *thrombolytic agents.* These drugs include streptokinase (Kabikinase), tissue plasminogen activator (abbre-viated as tPA, brand name Activase), and APSAC (Eminase). Although such medications increase the risk of internal bleeding, when administered during a heart attack, they can improve survival and have therefore become part of routine medical practice.

Postmenopausal hormone replacement therapy: Hormone replacement therapy (HRT) involves the use of the hormone estrogen, either alone or in combination with the female hormone progesterone. HRT was recommended for years as a way to prevent heart disease in older women on the basis of multiple observational studies that followed particular groups of women. These studies provided evidence that postmenopausal women taking HRT suffered fewer heart attacks and strokes, but it was never clear if HRT made the women healthier or if healthier women tended to take HRT. To clarify the role of HRT, the federal government launched a rigorous national study involving 16,000 women who were randomly assigned to take HRT or a placebo. After following the women for nearly seven years, researchers concluded that HRT causes a slight but significant increase in heart attacks, blood clots, and strokes as well as breast cancer. The consensus now is that HRT should not be taken to prevent heart disease. Even so, some women may choose to take HRT for a limited time to deal with menopause symptoms such as hot flashes and vaginal drying. The issue is complicated, so talk with your doctor if you are trying to decide whether to begin or how long to remain on HRT. (For more information, see another book in this series, *Healthy Women, Healthy Lives.*)

An alternative may be one of the so-called designer estrogens, known medically as selective estrogen receptor modulators (SERMs). These compounds bind with estrogen receptors and mimic the effects of estrogen in the body without causing some of the hormone's harmful effects. SERMs include medications such as raloxifene (Evista), which has been FDA-approved for osteoporosis, and tamoxifen (Nolvadex), used to treat breast cancer. Both also lower total cholesterol and "bad" LDL cholesterol, so they may be helpful for your heart. Some foods such as soybeans contain phytoestrogens, plant versions of the human hormone, and may help when consumed in sufficient quantities to reduce LDL cholesterol. (More on this in Chapter 6.)

Vitamins: The role of vitamin supplements in combating heart disease continues to be debated. Just five years ago, antioxidant vitamins, such as vitamin E, vitamin C, and beta-carotene, were hailed for reducing cardiovascular risk. Recently that theory has come into question. Studies with B vitamins have shown better results, although research in this area continues. The best bet, of course, is not to rely on vitamin supplements. Follow a healthy diet rich in fruits, vegetables, and whole grains. We'll discuss this in much greater detail in Chapters 6 and 7.

■ Medical Treatments

Coronary angioplasty and stent: This procedure, known medically as *percutaneous transluminal coronary angioplasty (PTCA)*, involves inserting a narrow tube known as a catheter into an artery in the groin and then threading it up to a narrowed artery in the heart. A flexible balloonlike section of the tube is then inflated to reopen the artery by pushing any accumulated plaque against the blood vessel wall. Once the arterial passage is cleared, the balloon is deflated. To keep the artery open, the cardiologist may also insert one or more stents, tiny mesh tubes, after which the catheter is removed.

This procedure, which is less invasive than heart surgery, can increase the supply of blood to the heart but does pose its own risks. The blood vessel wall may tear from the pressure of inflation. The plaque may rupture, spilling cholesterol-laden material into the blood vessel and increasing the risk that a blockage will develop downstream, elsewhere in the heart artery. About 17 to 40 percent of the time, stents may become clogged with scar tissue or additional plaque deposits after insertion, and the procedure may have to be repeated later.

■ Surgical Treatments

Coronary artery bypass: This surgical procedure can be used to treat angina or to prevent further damage caused by a heart attack. In the procedure, the surgeon harvests a vein or artery from somewhere else in the body and grafts it onto the aorta. The surgeon may use the saphenous veins, located in the legs, the internal mammary artery, located in the chest, or a radial artery from the forearm, and then redirect blood flow through the new artery—bypassing the blockage in the original artery. The operation can be lifesaving but also carries significant risks, among

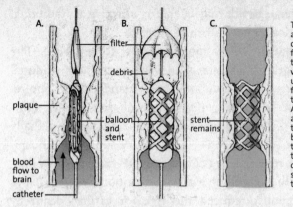

A.

B.

C.

filter

debris

plaque

balloon
and
stent

stent
remains

blood
flow to
brain

catheter

To catch small bits of plaque and other debris generated during angioplasty, a tiny filter can be attached to the tip of an angioplasty guide-wire (A). The physician unfurls the umbrella-like filter just before expanding the angioplasty balloon (B). As the balloon widens the arterial channel, the filter traps debris while allowing blood to pass through. Once the procedure is completed, the filter and balloon are deflated and removed; a stent may be left in place to keep the artery open (C).

Figure 11: **Insertion of a Stent**

them the risks involved with the operation itself (the mortality rate is 1 to 2 percent), risk for stroke caused by the surgery, and long-term mental decline following surgery.

Heart valve surgery: The heart has four valves that enable blood to exit the chamber properly. Most people who have valve defects are born with them, but if you have heart disease you may also de-velop a heart valve problem. If you do, surgery may be necessary to repair or replace the damaged valve with a mechanical prosthe-sis or a bioprosthesis (made of animal or donated human tissue).

■ Self-Help Strategies

Although the medications and surgical options we described can be helpful, none of them provides a magic bullet that will guaran-tee you a heart-healthy life. As we discussed earlier in the chapter, don't forget your head (and that wonderful brain inside) when you're thinking about your heart. The actions you take to help improve your own heart health may be just as effective as traditional medical and surgical options—if not more so.

Consider cardiac rehabilitation programs, for instance. The best of these programs combine supervised exercise, nutritional counseling, smoking cessation, and stress management. The research in these areas is compelling. A number of studies show that exercise and dietary changes following a heart attack actually slow the process of atherosclerosis and reduce subsequent hospitalizations. Other research has concluded that cardiac rehabilitation programs, which combine exercise, nutritional changes, and lifestyle modifications, reduced the risk for cardiac death by 25 percent. This reduction in mortality compares with that provided by medical interventions such as beta-blocker drugs and ACE inhibitors.

Stress management is another area that people too often ignore but that holds great potential for improving the health of your heart. A recent study by Duke researchers, for instance, found that teaching people with heart disease how to manage their stress significantly reduced their risk for further cardiac problems such as heart attacks, angioplasty, and bypass surgery. In fact, these researchers found that stress management was more helpful than medication, and slightly better than aerobic exercise, in reducing cardiac risk.

In the chapters that follow, we'll provide practical advice about how you can learn from this research and take steps to improve the health of your heart. This will include not only advice about nutrition, exercise, and stress management but also tips on how to become more mindful and peaceful as you go through life. We will explain how such mind/body interventions can reduce the symptoms and progression of heart disease—in many cases as effectively as medication or surgical interventions.

Change isn't easy, of course, but it may become easier if you think of it as an ongoing process. If you try to make a change and don't succeed, stop, take a breath, and try again. As the saying goes, the longest journey begins with the first step. And the first step may be simply deciding whether you're ready to change.

ARE YOU READY FOR A CHANGE?

You have to be ready to make a change, as you probably know instinctively. Drs. James Prochaska and Carlos DiClemente have pioneered a behavioral model that actually assesses how ready you are. We have adapted this model for use at the Mind/Body Medical Institute. To get started, ask yourself which of the statements below best describes your current state of mind. Each situation presented also identifies the type of resources you will need and suggests strategies.

- I've never thought about changing; I need information.
- I have thought about change but can't make a commitment yet.
- I want to change, but I need some motivation before I will do anything.
- I am trying to change, but I need support and would like to learn coping skills.
- I've made a change, but I find myself wavering and could use reinforcement.
- I made a change but then reverted to my old behavior; I need more motivation and support.

Chapter 3

Learn to Elicit the Relaxation Response

W HEN WE ARE THIRSTY, we drink. When we overexert ourselves, we rest. When we feel hungry, we eat. So why is it that when we feel stress we don't try to do something to relax? In our society, why do we assume that nonstop stress is a normal—rather than questionable—side of life?

Fortunately we have an inborn mechanism that can counterbalance the harmful effects of stress on our body, mind, and spirit. The mechanism triggers a physiological state known as the relaxation response, which can be elicited at will to create a state of profound peace and rest. The relaxation response may be difficult to elicit at first, but it will grow easier the more you practice. The results are worth the effort. Practiced on a regular basis, the relaxation response literally provides a soothing balm to your spirit—and your heart.

The relaxation response is so fundamental to wellness that it forms the foundation for all the programs offered through the Mind/Body Medical Institute, including the Cardiac Wellness Program.

■ The Fight-or-Flight Response

To appreciate the healing power of the relaxation response, you first have to understand another physiologic state that is its polar opposite: the fight-or-flight response. First described by Dr. Walter B. Cannon at Harvard Medical School in the 1920s, the fight-or-flight response evolved as a survival mechanism. When our ancient ancestors were confronted with a life-threatening situation (such as an approaching tiger), their bodies automatically shifted into a mode that enabled them to fight off the threat or flee for their lives.

Chances are, you have experienced your own version of an approaching tiger at least once. Perhaps you have stepped off a curb into a street and suddenly heard the screech of tires. You looked to your left, and seemingly out of nowhere a car was hurtling toward you, the wild-eyed driver desperately trying to stop. Do you remember how you felt at that moment or what you did? In all likelihood, within seconds, your heart started pounding in your chest, your muscles tensed, and without even thinking about it, you jumped out of the way. Perhaps you found yourself panting, struggling for breath as you reached the safety of the sidewalk. And these were only the changes you were aware of. Unbeknownst to you, your blood pressure and metabolism also increased dramatically along with your heart and breathing rates.

Fortunately in the modern world we don't routinely encounter life-threatening situations. What we tend to encounter, instead, are more mundane but still stressful events such as traffic jams and competing demands. The problem is, your brain does not distinguish between a life-threatening situation and routine stress. It perceives both in the same way. Even thinking about a stressful or threatening situation is enough to trigger the fight-or-flight response.

Most people activate the fight-or-flight response on a regular basis, largely as a result of encountering stressful events in the course of a normal day.

■ The Biology of Stress

The fight-or-flight response is a major component of a broader biological phenomenon, the stress response. Although we are still trying to determine the exact mechanisms involved, it is clear that stress triggers a cascade of hormones that contribute in various ways to heart disease. The word *hormone* is derived from the Greek word for *messenger,* and these chemicals are potent messengers indeed, conveying signals that create profound physiological changes throughout the body. Although hormones typically perform useful roles, they can become harmful in excessive amounts or when they circulate for extended periods.

When you encounter something stressful, the cerebral cortex, the part of your brain involved in consciousness, sends out a three-pronged alert to mobilize your body. Each of the three pathways involved in the stress response activates a particular set of resources that are essential to survival in the face of real danger.

One pathway involves the musculoskeletal system. A part of the brain known as the motor cortex sends signals directly to the muscles when a threat is perceived, increasing tension. As a result, muscles in the jaw, shoulders, and back tighten. You are physically braced to encounter a threat.

The second pathway is initiated when your cerebral cortex stimulates the hypothalamus, a part of the brain that helps regulate the two major components of the nervous system, the sympathetic nervous system (which tends to speed reactions up) and the parasympathetic nervous system (which slows them down). It's as if the hypothalamus is conducting triage, deciding where to direct the body's resources to fend off the perceived danger. In this way, the hypothalamus simultaneously mobilizes certain parts of the body to respond to a perceived threat while conserving the body's energy elsewhere.

As the sympathetic nervous system is activated, the hormones epinephrine (also known as adrenaline) and norepinephrine (nor-

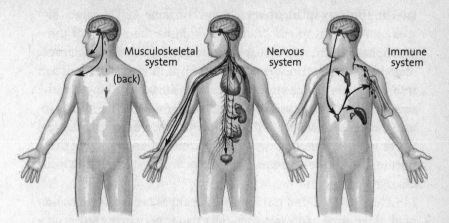

Musculoskeletal
system

(back)

Nervous
system

Immune
system

Figure 12: **The Stress Response**
When you become stressed, your brain activates three distinct pathways.

adrenaline) are released to rev things up. Heart rate, blood pressure, and the volume of blood being pumped out of the heart all increase. At the same time, the parasympathetic nervous system slows down other parts of the body by unleashing additional hormones that constrict certain blood vessels. Less blood reaches areas such as the skin and digestive organs, which are not needed for rapid response in an emergency. Blood flow is directed instead to the brain and muscles.

As the hypothalamus performs triage, directing energy to where it is most needed, you feel dramatic changes. Your heart starts pounding and your breathing becomes quick and shallow. You may even begin to sweat, as your body prepares to cool itself in the event you have to run away. You are probably less aware that the hormonal cascade has increased blood levels of glucose, cholesterol, and triglycerides to provide you with energy to fight, while preparing blood to clot more quickly in case you are injured. The problem, of course, is that this is the exact blood "profile" that increases the risk for a heart attack.

The third pathway is activated when the hypothalamus stimulates the pituitary gland to secrete the hormone ACTH, which signals another part of the brain and prompts the release of three additional hormones: cortisol, corticosterone, and aldosterone. Together, these hormones help boost immune system function into overdrive. If this hormonal rush is sustained, however, the immune system begins to wear out, compromising the body's internal defenses. We think this is why people who constantly feel stress, and are therefore exposed to a continuous cascade of these hormones, are more prone than others to illnesses such as heart disease.

Given the profound physiological changes caused by activation of all three stress pathways, it is clear that experiencing stress on a regular basis takes a toll. Our bodies just aren't meant to be in a constant state of arousal. To start, think of your response to a fire alarm being triggered over and over again. You can literally work yourself up into a state of hyperarousal in which your reactions to even the most minor of stresses (like waiting in a long line at a grocery store or driving in city traffic) put you in danger of having a heart attack.

Obviously, it's important to find ways to counteract the stress response so that we don't subject the heart to all that wear and tear. It is fortunate that the relaxation response, a natural mechanism, helps us do just that.

■ The Relaxation Response

The relaxation response is a physiological shift that puts the brakes on the runaway biological changes that first put us into overdrive. Eliciting the relaxation response leads to a quieting of the sympathetic nervous system. Your heartbeat and breathing return to normal. Oxygen consumption decreases and blood flows more easily throughout your body.

The electrical activity of the brain also changes during the relaxation response. When taken during the response, electroencephalogram (EEG) readings, which record brain wave activity, show an increase in frequency and intensity of alpha and theta slow brain waves in the cerebral cortex, the site of higher mental functions such as learning and memory. These types of brain waves are associated with a calm yet alert state of mind.

People who regularly elicit the relaxation response enjoy lasting effects that buffer their long-term sensitivity to stress. Faced with a threat, such people experience the same flood of stress hormones that we all do, but they don't react as strongly. One researcher, for instance, conducted a study in which he subjected volunteers to stress. He found that people who regularly elicited the relaxation response produced elevated levels of the hormone norepinephrine in response to stress, just as other volunteers did, but that their blood pressure and heart rate did not increase as much as the others' did.

We know *what* happens physiologically during the relaxation response, but we're still trying to determine *how* it happens. Although our research in this area continues, we think that a key molecular mechanism is nitric oxide. Despite being released only for short periods of time in the body, the effects of nitric oxide are long lasting. Among other things, nitric oxide contributes to the healthy functioning of the immune system, vascular system, and

---

TABLE 3

PHYSIOLOGICAL CHANGES COMPARED

	Fight-or-Flight Response	Relaxation Response
Metabolism	Increases	Decreases
Heart rate	Increases	Decreases
Blood pressure	Increases	Decreases
Breathing rate	Increases	Decreases
Muscle tension	Increases	Decreases

BENEFITS OF THE RELAXATION RESPONSE

- Reduction of physical symptoms related to stress
- Less anxiety; greater equanimity
- Less compulsive worrying, negative thinking, and self-criticism
- Better ability to concentrate and greater awareness
- More energy
- Self-acceptance
- Feeling of peace

---

brain. It also has antibacterial and antiviral properties that contribute to overall health. Probably its best-known role is as a vasodilator, an opener of blood vessels.

Based on research in our laboratory and by other scientists, we believe that when people elicit the relaxation response, they release nitric oxide. (This would explain the warming of the skin that typically occurs during the relaxation response—a sign of peripheral vasodilation.) We also speculate that this release of nitric oxide helps modify the artery-constricting effects of norepinephrine—thereby dampening a significant aspect of the stress response. (This would explain why people who elicit the relaxation response have elevated levels of norepinephrine but are resistant to its effects.) Finally, we believe that the relaxation response triggers the release of endorphins, natural painkillers that function much like morphine in the brain, which may explain why people experience a general sense of well-being after the shift.

Whatever its exact mechanisms, the benefits of eliciting the relaxation response are many. You will feel more focused and less distressed. It may feel odd at first to practice techniques used to elicit this response, much as it did when you tried to ride a bicycle or drive a car using a stick shift. But once you learn methods that

SIDEBAR 9

MONKS DEMONSTRATE THE AMAZING POWER OF THE MIND

Many of the physiological changes associated with the relaxation response are invisible to observers, although they can be measured with blood pressure monitors and EEGs. A group of monks provided a dramatic and visible example of the mind's power over the body. The monks, followers of Tibetan Buddhism, participate in a one-year period of visualization and meditation. Toward the end of this cycle, they sit naked in a cold room and wrap icy sheets around themselves. Using the power of their minds alone, the monks generate enough body heat to dry the sheets. Videotapes taken of these sessions show steam rising from the sheets as they dry—an amazing and quite visual testament to the power of mind over matter.

One of us, Dr. Benson, began collaborating with associates to study the monks more than twenty years ago. The team has recently begun a new study to measure physiological changes, for example, in metabolism and immune system function in an effort to better understand how the monks are able to generate such heat.

work for you, and practice them regularly, eliciting the relaxation response will become much easier.

■ Let Go . . . and Relax

You can best call forth the relaxation response, perhaps ironically, by letting go. You can't pursue the relaxation response the way you can pursue other goals, by jumping over a series of hurdles. To elicit the relaxation response, you lower barriers rather than jump over them, so that in effect relaxation comes to you. This is a different way of thinking for many people, who are unaware of the sheer volume of physical, mental, and emotional barriers they create every day.

Physical barriers: There are two physical barriers to relaxation: muscle tension and shallow chest breathing.

Muscle tension: Many people are so tense that their muscles never really relax. One sure sign of habitual tension, especially as you grow older, is the feeling of being stiff and creaky after sitting for a prolonged time. A specific sign is throwing your back out while putting groceries away. Or perhaps you develop trigger-point soreness in your neck and upper shoulders when working for long periods of time at a computer. Some muscle tightening is a natural consequence of aging; we all tend to become less limber with time. But other tightening has to do with the way stress affects the musculoskeletal system—putting us on the alert for rapid action. The problem is that your body begins to "remember" certain patterns of muscle tension and inclines toward them in response to stress.

It may surprise you to learn that using your muscles helps to solidify memories in the brain, but a long-standing body of research supports this notion. In the 1960s, a team of researchers reported that both animals and people who found their own way through a maze were better able to remember how they did so than their counterparts who were transported passively through the maze. Somehow the process of using the motor system helped to encode the memory. Additional research in how children learn to communicate finds that hand gestures seem to precede the development of language and arithmetic skills, as well as other types of mental activity.

If we accept the notion that muscle activity enhances memory, it then makes sense that certain physical postures may call up particular emotions or mental "attitudes." Simply put, assume a particular body posture or facial expression, and you are apt to trigger a mood. Research supports this. One study found that the act of smiling not only changed the position of facial muscles but also directly affected heart rate and breathing. Another researcher who studied facial muscle changes concluded that mood and muscles were part of a complex feedback loop that might perpetuate depression. And a participant involved in yet another study of facial positions said, "When my jaw was clenched and my brows down, I tried not to be angry but it just fit the position. I'm not in an angry mood, but I found my thoughts wandering to things that made me angry."

Although the relationship between the motor system and the mind is still under investigation, we are convinced that muscles matter when it comes to healing. Just as quieting the mind helps to quiet the body, so too does quieting the body help to relax the mind. We'll provide some details on how to let go of muscle tension later in this chapter.

Chest breathing: The way you breathe may pose another barrier to the relaxation response. Of course, everyone knows "how" to breathe or they wouldn't be alive. But it may surprise you to learn that there are two distinct ways of breathing and that one is much more conducive to relaxation than the other.

Most people are chest, or thoracic, breathers. If you breathe this way, your shoulders rise and chest expands as you inhale. Although your lungs do take in air, this is a relatively shallow way of breathing. And if you become tense, angry, or afraid, your breathing will tend to quicken, so that your breath comes in short staccato bursts. You may find yourself gasping, and your chest may feel constricted. Breathing this way all the time only fuels anxiety and tension.

A much healthier alternative is diaphragmatic, or abdominal, breathing. The diaphragm is a large, sheetlike muscle that covers the bottom of your lungs and is located above abdominal organs such as the stomach and liver. When you breathe diaphragmatically, your abdomen expands more than your chest. This is the way we breathe when we are born, but most of us switch to chest breathing by the time we are adults—either because of tension or the tendency to hold our stomachs in. That's a pity, because diaphragmatic breathing is a much more efficient way to breathe. The diaphragm adds muscle, literally, making each breath more powerful. When we breathe in, the diaphragm contracts so that more air is drawn into your lungs. When we exhale, the diaphragm relaxes and more air exits the lungs. Each breath draws in more life-sustaining oxygen, which helps to produce energy. As air is exhaled, we expel carbon dioxide wastes. By using our diaphragms to help us breathe, we get more benefit from each breath.

Diaphragmatic breathing indirectly helps the heart by reducing stress and calming our spirits. That's why deep breathing techniques are so central to our Cardiac Wellness Program. We'll provide tips on how to use diaphragmatic breathing to elicit the relaxation response later in this chapter.

SIDEBAR 10

TEST YOUR BREATHING

Are you a chest or diaphragmatic breather? Take this simple test to find out:

Sit in a comfortable position. Place one hand flat against your chest and the other against your abdomen. Now breathe in and out a few times. If the hand on your chest moves more than the hand on your abdomen, you're a chest breather. If the hand on your abdomen moves more than the hand on your chest, you're a diaphragmatic breather.

Mental barriers: Negative thoughts can pose a barrier to relaxation. How many times have you found your mind running at full speed, conjuring up worst-case scenarios or replaying old conflicts? It's as if we are programmed to think about things that have made us anxious or upset in the past, or that might happen in the future. Typically, thoughts that make you feel tense and stressed involve a perceived threat coupled with the feeling that you cannot cope with that threat. As a result, you tense up. To relax, you first have to let go of such negative thoughts.

Emotional barriers: Emotions can also act as a barrier to relaxation. Troubling emotions often surface when you are faced with the hassles of everyday life, such as a long line at the bank when you have only ten minutes to spare or a copy machine that breaks down when you need to meet a deadline. What do you feel in such circumstances? Do you become angry and anxious, or do you let the inconvenience roll off your back and come up with an alternative plan? If you tend toward negative emotional reactions, then you are likely adding to your overall tension and creating a barrier to relaxation. Strive for more equanimity. We'll show you how.

■ How to Elicit the Relaxation Response

Given the physical, mental, and emotional barriers we've just described, you may find it daunting at first to elicit the relaxation response. Fortunately, a number of techniques will help, and we will describe them briefly in the pages that follow. Experiment until you find the method that works for you. Many people also find that combining techniques is the best way to go.

The following general guidelines will help you as you elicit the relaxation response, no matter which method (or combination of methods) you choose.

Start your day with relaxation: It's best to elicit the relaxation response first thing in the morning. This starts the day off by easing your mind and body, so that you will be less reactive to the stresses and hassles you will undoubtedly encounter. Many people find it ideal to spend twenty minutes practicing before breakfast, before the rest of the household is awake. If you just aren't a morning person, try to take time before lunch or dinner. But if you must miss that morning session, try to do a "mini" relaxation response for five minutes whenever you can find the time. You will find that this provides a sense of peace and awareness that will serve you well later in the day. (For more on "minis," see pages 87 to 89.)

Find a peaceful place: Find or create a special place where you can elicit the relaxation response without worrying about being interrupted by a ringing telephone, the sounds of the television, or family members running in and out. If you don't have an entire room you can use, locate a quiet corner somewhere. All it may take is rearranging some furniture and perhaps adding a few objects, such as a plant or a picture of a peaceful scene, to set the tone. Once you identify a spot that works for you, return to it every day. As you associate your special place with relaxation, you may find that just returning every day will help you to calm down.

Get comfortable: You can elicit the relaxation response in any position that makes you comfortable, as long as it isn't so relaxing that you fall asleep. Most people prefer to sit in a well-padded chair. You can also sit on a big floor pillow or lie down on your back. If you're using movement, such as hatha yoga, you may even stand. Whatever posture you choose, remember that clothing also matters. Wear loose-fitting shirts and slacks, and go barefoot or wear socks so as not to constrain your feet.

Practice regularly: To obtain the most benefit from the relaxation response, elicit it regularly. We recommend practicing once a day for twenty minutes or twice a day for ten minutes at a time. In this way, you will attune your body to periodic relaxation, regularly lower your blood pressure and heart rate, and provide a buffer against the stress hormones circulating in your bloodstream. To avoid worrying about the time, set an egg timer, clock, or watch for your desired number of minutes. You can place the alarm in another room, or cover it with a pillow, so that it won't startle you when it goes off.

Focus, focus, focus: Focusing your mind is a continual process. If you are like most people, you will find it hard at first to quiet your mind's internal dialogue and random thoughts. As soon as you do, it may seem as if your brain fills with static. That's why all the relaxation response techniques involve some type of repetitive focus—the breath, a sound, word, or phrase repeated silently or aloud.

Of course, most people who are new to the relaxation response find that their minds do not switch off easily. You may find that you are distracted by thoughts that seem to bubble up from nowhere. This is natural. The challenge is to let the thoughts come, and then let them go. Don't dwell on them. That is where our last general guideline, a passive attitude, comes in.

A passive attitude: We live in such an action-oriented world, this step may be difficult at first. A passive mental attitude is one that is accepting, not judgmental. So as you elicit the relaxation response, try not to evaluate what's happening or berate yourself if you're not relaxing fast enough. Just breathe, focus your mind, and let other thoughts come and go as if they were actors walking onstage and you were in the audience, watching. Accept whatever arises—thoughts, feelings, images, sensations, or external noise.

This may be difficult at first, but it becomes easier with time. You will begin to step back mentally and allow yourself to be an observer of or witness to your thoughts rather than a judge. When you find yourself thinking everyday thoughts, simply return to your mental focus. Then let the thoughts subside. Or label

---

SIDEBAR 11

TECHNIQUES TO ELICIT THE RELAXATION RESPONSE

- Diaphragmatic breathing
- Meditation
- Imagery or visualization
- Body scan
- Progressive muscle relaxation
- Mindfulness
- Autogenic training
- Yoga
- Tai Chi (see Chapter 8)
- Repetitive exercise (see Chapter 8)

---

thoughts as they appear (work, family) and imagine putting them in a box.

Above all, don't try too hard. Remember that in order to elicit the relaxation response you need to let go. That includes letting go of expectations and goals. Try not to compare one session with another; every relaxation response experience is different. Enjoy the variations!

■ Specific Techniques

Diaphragmatic breathing: The breath is a simple yet powerful technique you can use to elicit the relaxation response. We've found in follow-up surveys that our patients use breathing techniques to deal with stress more consistently than they use other relaxation methods.

You may think at first that it's impossible to learn how to breathe differently. But the breath is actually one of the only physiological functions that is both voluntary and involuntary in nature. That means we can learn how to modulate our breathing to reduce stress and induce calm. Try this exercise to become more aware of the way you breathe now, and gradually shift to diaphragmatic breathing.

1. Wear comfortable, loose-fitting clothing. Lie down on the floor if it's comfortable, or sit in a chair with your buttocks near the edge while keeping your back straight.
2. Place one hand on your chest and the other on your abdomen, just above your belly button. Take a deep breath. Your lower hand should move more than the hand on your chest. Concentrate on drawing air down into your abdomen until your belly rises and falls with each breath.
3. Breathe through your nose rather than your mouth; this will warm the breath, filter air, and enable you to breathe more deeply.

If you have trouble at first, don't worry. As long as you're breathing, you're headed in the right direction! It sometimes helps to imagine the lungs as balloons that fill with air and then deflate. Other people find that it helps to feel the rhythm of their breath, as if they were watching waves washing ashore: gentle breath rolling in; gentle breath rolling out. A third technique is to imagine that you are blowing out a candle. Inhale deeply through the nose and then exhale with your lips rounded and mouth open slightly. Feel free to make noise as you exhale, either by blowing out air or by sighing as you release it.

Continue this abdominal breathing for at least five to ten breaths, and longer if you feel you enjoy the relaxation. (If you feel dizzy at any time, discontinue the deep breathing immediately and return to normal breathing until you feel better.) As you end your breathing session, take a deep breath and slowly open your eyes. Sometimes people feel a little light-headed, so move slowly until your sense of balance returns. You will probably feel much calmer than you did before you started.

Meditation: The word *meditation* may bring to mind an image of a Hindu priest sitting cross-legged on a cushion. That is one position in which to meditate, but there are others. In addition, we can all meditate, no matter what culture we were born into. It is simply a matter of learning to turn our attention inward rather than paying attention to what is going on in the world around us.

Usually we do exactly the opposite of meditating, of course. Think about the last time you were dealing with a customer or sitting in a meeting. You were probably trying to listen to the person talking while tuning out other sounds, like those of a colleague clearing his throat or a child crying. And if you were bored at the meeting and found your mind drifting, you might have caught yourself and refocused on the speaker. It's the same thing with meditation, except the focus is directed inward. Try the following steps to practice meditation.

1. Find a quiet and comfortable place to sit. A well-padded chair will do, although many people like to sit on a big, flat pillow.
2. Take a few deep diaphragmatic breaths to calm your mind and body.
3. Concentrate on your mental focus, such as a neutral word or phrase that you repeat silently to yourself.
4. If your personal thoughts or something from the outside world distracts you, take a deep breath and return to your mental focus—as if you were directing your attention back to a speaker in the room. Instead of getting caught up in an internal dialogue, gently redirect your attention to your breath, focus word, or phrase. You will find that with time and practice, this becomes easier.
5. Continue for ten to twenty minutes. (Place a clock nearby so that when your time is up you can glance over and then choose to continue or stop.)
6. Take a few deep breaths, stretch, and slowly stand up.

FOCUS WORDS AND PHRASES

Listed below are words you can use to focus your mind. You may think of others, of course. The idea is to find words that convey feelings of peace, spirituality, and acceptance.

Neutral
Calm
Let go
Let it be
Love
My time
Ocean
Oh well
One
Peace
Relax

Christian
Come, Lord
Hail Mary
Lord, have mercy
Lord Jesus Christ, have mercy
    on me

Our Father
Our Father, who art in heaven
The Lord is my shepherd

Jewish
The Lord is my shepherd
Echad ("One")
Hashem ("The Name")
Shalom ("Peace")
Sh'ma Yisroel ("Hear, O Israel")

Eastern
Om (the universal sound)
Shantih ("Peace")

Islamic
Allah

Words to Avoid
Words that sound like commands or are normally used in expressing harsh emotions do not make good focus words. Choose words like these, and you may find your blood pressure rising, not falling.

Go
Hurry

Now
Stop

Imagery and visualization: When you dream, or when you close your eyes and remember something, you create a mental image that does not exist in a physical sense. Some images can be frightening (as those that cause a nightmare) and others comforting (a fond memory). Images affect us physically and emotionally; our mind reacts to a mental image in the same way as it would to a physical object or event.

You can harness the power of visualization in order to elicit the relaxation response. We use a number of guided imagery scenarios in the Cardiac Wellness Program. All involve imagining a setting that is peaceful or comforting and then focusing your mind on it as it unfolds. Allow all your senses to be present to your experience. Sometimes people can do this on their own, as when they imagine taking a walk on the beach. Others find it helpful to listen to a tape. (For more information, see Appendix 3: Organizations and Resources.)

Try this short visualization exercise about a safe place, which is one of our most popular.

1. Assume a comfortable position, either sitting in a chair or lying down.
2. Imagine a beautiful light centered in the focus of your breathing. As you look into the light, you notice a scene developing that you recognize as having special meaning to you. It is a safe place, a place where you feel comfortable, relaxed, and at peace. It could be a place you remember from your childhood, a place you know as an adult, or an imaginary place that you create to provide yourself with security and comfort.
3. Allow yourself to settle in to this safe place. Find a comfortable position and let your body relax. Let your senses take in the surroundings. What do you see, what do you smell, what do you hear, what do you feel? Your awareness is focused on being with yourself, feeling safe and at peace.
4. If you notice your mind drifting toward thoughts or concerns of the past or future, note these thoughts without judgment,

then gently let them go, take a deep breath, and bring your awareness back to your safe place. Use your breath, or a repeated word or phrase, to anchor your awareness in the moment as you settle in to the comfort and peacefulness of this special, safe place. Continue to rest quietly for the next several minutes.

5. When you feel ready, slowly shift your awareness out from your safe place to the external attributes of the room. Before you leave your special place, pay attention to how the safety and security felt, free of stress and conflict. That way, when you recognize increasing stress in your everyday life, you will have the memory of feeling peaceful and quiet and the ability to shift your thoughts to a safe place in the present moment.

6. Begin to pay attention to the sensations you experience. Open your eyes, stretch, and begin to move in a slow, gentle manner, noting how it feels to move. Watch your thoughts as you transition back to the external world.

Another visualization exercise involves a beach. See if it makes you feel more relaxed.

1. Sit in a quiet place.
2. Close your eyes and take a few deep diaphragmatic breaths. Breathe in a feeling of peace and relaxation, and breathe out tension and stress. Don't force your breathing, just notice its rhythm.
3. Now imagine yourself standing on a staircase twenty steps above a beautiful beach. Walk down a few steps, becoming aware of the sand under your feet.
4. Take a few more steps and become aware of the breeze on your shoulders.
5. As you reach the tenth step, you begin to feel the sun against your back.
6. A few more steps, and you hear the waves washing gently ashore.
7. When you get to the bottom stair, step onto the sand and

slowly walk toward the water. Be aware of all your senses—the sights, smells, sounds, and sensations.

8. As you reach the water, notice its color, the sound of the waves, the feel of sand under your feet. Feel the sun against your skin and a breeze against your face.
9. Walk slowly up and down the beach, noting all sensations.
10. After ten minutes, take a last slow look at the water, then walk back toward the stairs.
11. Walk up one step at a time, noting the experience of the beach fading into your memory with each step.
12. At the top of the stairs, slowly return your focus to the sounds around you in the room.

Body scan: You can also become more in tune with your body, and relax in the process, by doing a body scan. This technique helps you to focus on one part of your body at a time, releasing any tension you feel there. You can practice a body scan using the steps below.

1. Start by taking a few deep diaphragmatic breaths to quiet your mind and body.
2. Bring your awareness to your right big toe. Think of your toe as being made of atoms, with space between the atoms, so that the toe feels open and spacious.
3. Now shift your focus to your second, third, fourth, and fifth toes.
4. Gradually shift your awareness to the ball of your foot, then the arch, top of your foot, ankle, calf, knee, thigh, and hip. As you shift your awareness, continue to visualize the atoms and space between the atoms.
5. Allow your whole right leg to relax into the support of the floor, feeling open, spacious, and light.
6. Repeat steps 2 through 5 with your left foot and leg.
7. Now bring your awareness to your back, and notice each ver-

tebra, one at a time, seeing the space around the vertebra as open and spacious, relaxing all the muscles in your back.

8. Shift your awareness to your abdomen and your chest, seeing the space between all your organs and relieving any restrictions that might be there. Allow your abdomen to feel spacious and light.

9. Bring your awareness to your right thumb, second, third, fourth, and fifth fingers. Then shift your attention to the palm of your hand, wrist, forearm, elbow, upper arm, and shoulder. Feel your whole right arm as open, spacious, and light.

10. Repeat step 9 with your left hand and arm.

11. Now bring your awareness to your neck and jaw. Yawn. Allow your jaw to relax. Become aware of your eyes, allowing them to rest gently in their sockets. Then shift your attention to your forehead, softening the muscles of your jaw, at the top of your head, and at the back of your head.

12. Let your whole body rest softly into the support of the floor. Bring your awareness to your breath. As you inhale, imagine bringing energy and light into your body, and as you exhale, release any tension you may still be holding in your body.

13. If you notice that any part of your body is still tense, focus your breathing in that area, releasing tension each time you exhale. If your mind wanders, simply acknowledge the thoughts and gently return to your focus.

14. Take a few minutes to notice the experience of yourself when your mind is quiet and body relaxed.

15. Now it's time to bring your awareness back to the room. Slowly open your eyes. Take deep breaths. Stretch and yawn if you would like to.

Another body scan we recommend, "Open Your Heart," is particularly suited to people with heart disease. Our patients find that this body scan not only helps them to elicit the relaxation response but also focuses healing energy on the heart.

1. Find a comfortable position, lying on a mat or the floor.

2. Focus on your breath. Take a few slow, deep breaths. Feel your belly slowly rise as you inhale and slowly fall as you exhale. Let your body begin to relax.

3. Now bring your awareness to the top of your head. Breathe in a feeling of warmth and relaxation. Let the back of your head gently relax against the mat or floor. Let your eyes gently close, as any tension around the forehead or eyes begins to melt away. Feel the warmth and relaxation settling into your cheeks and jaw.

4. Slowly bring your awareness to the back of your neck and shoulders. Let your neck and shoulders relax. Let your arms feel warm and relaxed by your side.

5. Bring your awareness to your chest, to your "heart center." Focus on your emotional heart, the place where you hold love and compassion. Visualize your heart as a bud, a flower waiting to bloom. Is this your emotional heart? Is your heart closed? Have you built walls around your heart to protect yourself?

6. Now visualize your heart as a beautiful flower in bloom, and focus on it. Allow your heart to be open to love, compassion, and forgiveness. Let go of uncertainty and doubt. Let the walls you have built around your heart begin to melt away. Breathe in love and compassion. Like the flower, allow your heart to feel the warmth and healing rays of the sun.

7. Now visualize your physical heart as strong and healthy. The arteries are open and nourishing your heart muscle. Your heartbeat is slow and regular. Your blood pressure is normal. Your whole upper torso is warm and relaxed.

8. Bring your awareness to your middle and lower spine. Breathe in warmth and relaxation. Let go of tension. Feel the rise and fall of your belly with each breath. Bring your awareness to any area of your abdomen that might need additional healing.

9. Focus your attention on your lower extremities. Let your legs

relax totally into the support of the floor. Breathe warmth and relaxation into your hips, thighs, calves, and feet. Let any tension you are aware of begin to melt away. Your whole body is now totally relaxed. Breathe in warmth and breathe out tension.

10. For the next few minutes, focus your attention back on your heart. Breathe in a sense of appreciation or love for yourself or others. Feel your heart open and relax. Remain in this peaceful place for the next few minutes.

11. When you are ready, you can slowly begin the transition back to being aware of the room around you. Begin to deepen your breathing. Stretch or yawn slowly, as though awakening from a wonderful rest.

12. Slowly open your eyes. You may wish to roll on your side and bring your knees to your chest. Allow yourself to take in the quiet of the moment. Feel how relaxed and peaceful you are. When you are ready, you can sit up slowly. Go about the rest of your day feeling relaxed and refreshed.

Progressive muscle relaxation: As we mentioned earlier in this chapter, your muscles may be chronically tense. Although the diaphragmatic breathing techniques we described should help you lose some of this muscle tension, you have another option, known as progressive muscle relaxation. The idea of this technique is to tense and then release large muscle groups, such as your shoulders, biceps, and thighs, in a sequential fashion. You might start at the top of your body and work your way downward, or vice versa. Not only does this help you to relax, by releasing the muscle tension, but it also reminds you that you are in control of the tension. And as you relax physically, you will find that you also relax mentally and emotionally.

Try this short exercise in progressive muscle relaxation.

1. Sit in a comfortable position in a quiet place.
2. Close your eyes.

3. Begin the muscle relaxation sequence starting with your feet. To do this, extend your legs in front of you. Pull your feet back, tilting your toes toward your knees.

4. Feel what the tension is like and location of the sensation. Relax and take a deep breath. (Repeat this for steps 5 through 12.)

5. Tense the muscles of your thighs as if you were trying to lift your legs against a weight.

6. Pinch your buttocks in and up, making them hard, as if you were seated upon a rock.

7. Pull your abdomen in, hardening it.

8. Pull your hands back at the wrists, tilting them toward your elbows.

9. Clench your fists.

10. Raise your shoulders up to your ears.

11. Grin, clenching your teeth tightly.

12. Raise your eyebrows and pinch them together.

13. Now take five slow deep breaths through your nose. Allow the breath to fill your abdomen, then exhale slowly. Then let your breath come on its own; watch your breath coming in and going out.

14. Continue doing a breath focus as in step 13 for ten to twenty minutes. When you finish, stay quiet for several minutes, at first with your eyes closed and then with them open. Notice the contrast between how you feel now versus how you felt at the beginning of the relaxation exercise. Allow yourself to adjust slowly to your surroundings.

Mindfulness: This is a handy technique if you feel as though you are so busy you have no time to meditate or sit down and do a progressive muscle relaxation. Mindfulness involves focusing on one task at a time and trying to really appreciate all aspects of that task. It may help to pick a task you normally consider boring, such as washing the dishes or weeding the garden. You can focus on the ingredients as you cook dinner or the motion your body makes as you walk or dance. The idea is to be aware of everything you see, hear, smell, touch, and taste during the activity—in other words, be open to the full sensory experience.

Try this: eat a raisin mindfully. Start by picking just one raisin out of a box. Hold it in the palm of your hand and look at the raisin's color and texture. Roll it between two fingers to see how firm it is, to feel its bumpy surface. Holding it up to your nose, inhale to enjoy the aroma. Now place the raisin in your mouth and roll it around on your tongue as if you were tasting fine wine. Finally chew the raisin slowly, taking in the flavor and texture.

By focusing on a particular task, you become present "in the moment." This means that you are not reliving something that has already happened or anticipating or worrying about something that has not yet happened. In this way, you may find that your body and mind relax. Since stress largely involves perception, reducing stress can be as simple as changing your attitude while performing a routine task or getting through an everyday hassle. Instead of being annoyed at the time it is taking, try to savor the sensations of the experience. Notice what you learn about yourself in the process. You may be surprised at how much you begin to enjoy tasks you once dreaded.

Autogenic training: Autogenic training involves a series of brief phrases that focus your attention on various parts of your body and help convey how you want to feel. The goal is to consciously rebalance your cardiovascular and respiratory systems so that you will feel more relaxed. Try this exercise to understand how autogenic training works.

1. Sit in a quiet and warm place (75 to 80 degrees Fahrenheit).
2. Slowly and silently repeat the following phrases to yourself: I am beginning to feel quiet. I am beginning to feel relaxed. My feet, knees, and hips feel heavy. Heaviness and warmth are

flowing through my feet and legs. My hands, arms, and shoulders feel heavy. Warmth and heaviness are flowing through my arms, hands, and fingertips. My neck, jaw, tongue, and forehead feel relaxed and smooth. My whole body feels quiet, heavy, and comfortable. I am comfortable and relaxed. My breathing is slow and regular. I am aware of my calm, regular heartbeat. My mind is becoming quieter as I focus inward. I feel still. Deep in my mind I experience myself as relaxed, comfortable, and still. I am alert in a quiet, inward way.

3. Now finish your relaxation and begin to take several deep diaphragmatic breaths as you say the following phrases to yourself: As I finish my relaxation, I take in several deep, reenergizing breaths, bringing light and energy into every cell of my body.

Yoga: For thousands of years, people around the world have practiced yoga to bring the mind, body, and spirit into harmony. There are many types of yoga practices, and many of these can be used to elicit the relaxation response. In the Cardiac Wellness Program, we tend to use hatha yoga. This practice involves coordinating movement with the breath while moving in and out of postures, or *asanas*, to release body tension and quiet the mind. While holding certain postures, you also employ breathing techniques in order to release body tension and deepen relaxation. If you are new to yoga, or haven't stretched your muscles in a while, you might want to try Iyengar yoga. In this type of yoga, the postures are performed while supporting yourself with chairs, pillows, and other objects. Kundalini yoga combines postures with visualizations, soft chanting, and meditation. Kripalu yoga involves a continuous series of spontaneous movements that are combined with meditation. We do not recommend ashtanga or "power" yoga, which involves more difficult postures (some of which may even increase blood pressure) and an emphasis on building strength and stamina rather than cultivating an attitude of relaxation.

Think for a moment about how you feel when you yawn, which is a natural way to release tension. Yoga is much like a fancy yawn for your whole body. By practicing various postures that are steady and comfortable, we can learn where we are holding tension in our bodies and move in ways to provide release.

Research on yoga shows that it is useful in improving psychological and physical health. Various studies have found that regular yoga practice improves cardiovascular circulation, digestion, respiration, immune system functioning, and increases flexibility and muscle tone. Yoga also reinforces the idea that you can maintain a basic "resting state" in your body even while going about your daily activities.

We've included a few sample yoga postures that can be done alone, or in a series, so that you can get a flavor for this discipline. To learn more, you may find it helpful to join a class or watch a videotape.

Sun salute: A great way to get started is to do the sun salute. The traditional sun salute is a series of twelve yoga postures in which movement is coordinated with breathing. Because this traditional series may prove too difficult for people new to yoga, we recommend that you start with a modified version of the sun salute. With practice, you may be able to do these postures as if they were part of one fluid movement. As its name implies, the sun salute was traditionally done in the morning, facing the east as the sun rose. You can do the following modified practice while sitting or standing. Our patients find it easier to perform than the traditional version, which involves several deep bends and spine stretches that require a high degree of balance and flexibility. The modified version enables you to open yourself up and draw energy from the universe without hurting yourself.

1. Bring your hands together in front of you at the level of your heart in the prayer position, with palms pressed lightly together. Elbows should be bent and roughly parallel to your hands.

2. Now reach out in front of you, inhaling slowly as you do so, with your palms down.

3. Stretch your arms outward, on either side of you, as you exhale and relax your shoulders.

4. Bring your arms back to the center, palms still facing downward, as you inhale.

5. Now clasp your hands back in the prayer position as you exhale, and draw your arms back toward your body.

6. Repeat steps 2 and 3, keeping shoulders relaxed and stretching your arms, releasing tension through your fingertips.

7. With your arms still extended on either side of you, turn your palms upward as you inhale. Imagine you are balancing a ball in each palm; feel the weight. Exhale.

8. Now raise your arms slowly over your head, inhaling, until your fingertips touch and you form a circle with your arms. Exhale.

9. Breathe deeply, then exhale as you press your palms together over your head, hands in the prayer position.

10. Bring your arms down in front of you, hands still pressed together in the prayer position, as if you were pulling energy downward into your heart.

11. Continue the downward motion, as your hands sink below chest level and then naturally part. Release the energy.

12. Breathe in deeply as your arms and hands rest at your sides (if standing) or on your lap (if sitting).

Cat pose: Now get down on your hands and knees, facing the floor. This is a great position for releasing tension in your back and throughout your body. It is similar to the kinds of stretches that cats do instinctively to keep so limber.

1. Keep your arms straight and rest on your hands and knees. Your knees should be under your hips and your hands directly under your shoulders.

2. Slowly inhale as you lift your head up so that you can look to-

ward the ceiling, as you simultaneously let your lower back sag so that your tailbone reaches upward and your belly extends downward.

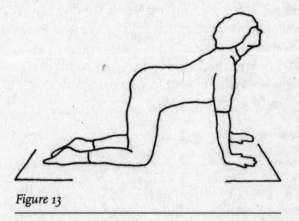

Figure 13

3. Now slowly exhale as you tuck your chin in toward your chest, round your back, and pull your belly inward.

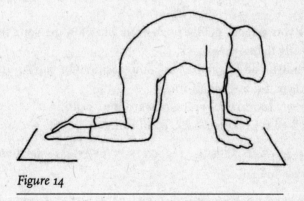

Figure 14

4. Repeat slowly several times, synchronizing the movement of your spine with your breathing. The more slowly and focused you are, the more effective your stretch will be.

Child pose: This can be done right after the cat pose, and is intended to make you feel safe and secure.

1. Sit back on your heels.
2. Lean forward while reaching to touch the floor, until your forehead is resting comfortably on the floor. (You can use a towel or blanket to cushion your head.) Your torso should be resting on your thighs.
3. Pull your arms backward so that your hands come to rest behind you, parallel to your feet, as you exhale slowly to release tension from your shoulders.

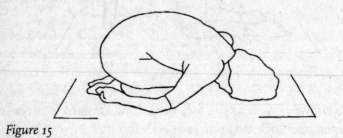

Figure 15

4. As you exhale, gently push your hips toward your feet and gently flatten your back.
5. While breathing slowly, hold the position for half a minute, or longer if it feels comfortable.
6. Slowly round your spine upward into a sitting position.
7. Roll gently on your back, continuing to breathe abdominally.

Knee to chest: This is a good way to release tension from muscles.

1. Lie on your back on the floor, using a mat if necessary for comfort.
2. Bend your knees so that your feet are flat on the floor, close to your buttocks and slightly apart.

3. As you exhale, slowly bring your right knee to your chest. You can wrap your hands around the outside of your knee.

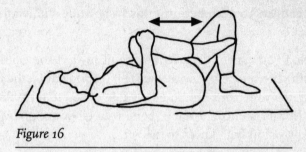

Figure 16

4. Now slowly move the same leg a few inches away from your chest as you inhale.
5. Slowly repeat this gentle back-and-forth motion six times, synchronizing the movement of your leg with your breathing.
6. Repeat steps 3 through 5 with your left leg, exhaling as you draw your knee to your chest and inhaling as you extend your leg outward.
7. Repeat six times and rest.
8. Grasp both knees and draw your legs slowly toward your chest, exhaling as you do so. Feel the movement of your spine as your knees come closer to your chest, and let go of the tension in your hips.

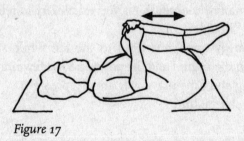

Figure 17

9. Move your knees clockwise in a circular direction to massage your spine. (You may reverse direction and go counterclockwise if you want to.)

10. Inhale slowly as you stretch your legs back toward the floor.
11. Repeat several times and rest.

Spinal twist: You can perform this twist while still lying on the floor.

1. Bend your knees so that they point toward the ceiling and bring them together, with your feet resting flat on the floor.
2. Stretch your arms out on either side of you to form the letter *T.* (If this is uncomfortable, bend your elbows slightly.)
3. Slowly shift both knees to the left.

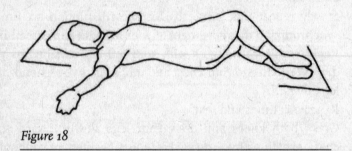

Figure 18

4. Slowly turn your head right to look in the opposite direction. You should feel a gentle stretch in your chest and spine.
5. Rest for a few moments. As you exhale, try to release tension in your shoulders.
6. Now slowly turn your head to the left while shifting both knees to the right. Hold the position for a few moments while inhaling and exhaling slowly and deeply.
7. Repeat several times.

■ Common Obstacles to Practice

Over the years, as we've instructed people in how to elicit the relaxation response, we've also noticed that most people meet the same obstacles in their practice. Fortunately, all can be dealt with in some way.

Not enough time: If you are pressed for time and feel like you can't possibly fit in twenty minutes a day, that may be one of the reasons you have heart disease. Look at your schedule closely. Is there anything that you can drop? If not, try getting up earlier in the morning. Or try two ten-minute sessions sometime during the day. It's worth it. Practice the relaxation response regularly, and you will begin to feel more energized and less frazzled. So just do it!

Can't settle down: If you find that you are jittery and restless, try doing some hatha yoga stretching, go for a short walk, or take a warm bath or shower.

You fall asleep: Some people fall asleep while eliciting the relaxation response, especially if they are lying down on the floor or a mat. If this happens to you, try sitting upright so that your head and neck are erect. That way, if you nod off, you'll feel yourself falling asleep. Another possibility is that you are practicing at a time of day when you are too tired to focus. Try practicing at a different time. Finally, try not to practice the relaxation response after a big meal, which will only make you feel tired.

External distractions: A dog barking, your children fighting, a telephone ringing. Unless you practice the relaxation response in a soundproof booth, you will hear some external noise during your practice session. Try wearing earplugs or headphones to muffle the sounds. Or visualize the noises as becoming smaller and receding into the horizon. As you exhale, imagine pushing the noises away.

Racing thoughts: When your body quiets down, does it seem as though your mind speeds up? This is where you'll benefit by assuming a passive stance. Understand that your mind was made to think and it is just doing what comes naturally. Then let the thoughts go. You may find it helpful to imagine the thoughts as clouds passing by.

Fear and anxiety: Sometimes people find that as they quiet their bodies and try to focus their minds, they become panicky and anxious. This may have something to do with the fear of letting down barriers or opening yourself to a new experience. If this happens to you, open your eyes and find a spot or point to focus your attention on. Take a few deep diaphragmatic breaths. Use visualization if necessary to imagine a warm, safe place. Usually fear and anxiety will pass with time, as you practice the relaxation response more frequently.

Revisit painful memories: Sometimes as you elicit the relaxation response, you may find yourself confronting things that happened in the past. These memories can evoke strong emotions. As with racing thoughts, the best strategy is to acknowledge the resurfacing of these memories but then to let them go rather than dwelling on them. Inhale and exhale deeply. It may also help to write in a journal about these events and emotions. (See Chapter 5 for information on dealing with emotions.) If troubling memories continue to occur, you may need to discuss them with a mental health professional or counselor.

"I'm not doing it right": There is no right or wrong way when it comes to the relaxation response; that's why we've suggested a number of techniques to elicit it and have encouraged you to experiment, to find which one works for you. If you are able to relax even a little, then you are making progress. Every step toward relaxation is a step in the right direction. Let go of judgments and just notice the experience as it unfolds.

Fear of "letting go": If you find yourself relaxing so much that you feel as though you are sinking or that your breath has stopped, this may scare you at first. Actually, it's a sign that you have begun to elicit the relaxation response in a very deep way. Remember that you can always open your eyes if you feel anxious. It will take some time to get used to the feeling of "letting go."

Body feels different: During a practice session, you may notice that your hands or feet begin to tingle or that your arms and legs feel heavy. This is actually a sign that you have begun to relax. Try to experience and enjoy the new sensations rather than be distracted by them.

■ Mini-Relaxation Exercises

Mini-relaxation responses are a bit like booster shots for the soul. They are miniature versions of techniques used to elicit the relaxation response and generally take only a minute or so to do. "Minis," as we commonly refer to them, can involve taking a few deep diaphragmatic breaths or doing gentle stretches to relieve tension. Minis are useful for helping you to stay in the present moment and extend the benefits of the relaxation response throughout the day; for example, when stuck in traffic on the way to work or having to deal with a difficult customer.

Minis work best if you do them in conjunction with regular practice of eliciting the relaxation response. In this way, you start your day off in a calm frame of mind and the minis enable you to remain focused and relaxed throughout the day.

You can do mini-relaxation exercises any time during the day and in virtually any location: your car, a bus, the office, or while doing errands on the way home. You can also use minis to deal with stressful situations, such as a visit to the dentist's office.

Some of our patients find it helpful to use the "blue dot"

SAMPLE MINI-RELAXATION EXERCISES

Mini version 1: When caught in a traffic jam, release physical tension by doing a few short exercises. Slowly roll your head forward, then backward, then to one side and the other. Drop your shoulders and loosen your grip on the steering wheel. Stretch your fingers out and wiggle them. Take a few deep diaphragmatic breaths while repeating a mantra. (For example: Say "I am" while inhaling and "at peace" while exhaling.)

Mini version 2: Feeling tense? Sit quietly in a chair for a few minutes. Take a deep diaphragmatic breath, and as you exhale, say the number *ten* to yourself. Inhale again, and when you exhale, say *nine*. Continue until you reach zero.

Mini version 3: Breathe deeply and slowly. As you inhale, count silently from one to four. Then as you exhale, count backward (four, three, two, one). Repeat several times. The counting will help you to slow your breathing and focus your mind.

Mini version 4: During a routine daily task, try to pay attention to what is going on both around you and within you. For example, as you walk to work, pay attention to the other people on the street. Notice the sky; is it cloudy? Blue? Are birds chirping? Are any flowers budding? Feel the rhythm of your body as you walk and try to breathe deeply, even if it means slowing your pace.

Mini version 5: Take a few moments every day to stop the routine. If you work in an office, take a walk to the watercooler or around the halls to stretch your legs. Look out your window and notice what is going on in the area outside your office. Or if the weather is nice, go outside for a few minutes to get some fresh air.

---

method to remind themselves to do mini-relaxation exercises throughout the day. You can buy small adhesive dots in any office supply store. We like blue because it's a restful color, but you can certainly pick whatever color appeals to you. (Try, however, to avoid loud colors such as red or orange, which tend to project energy, not re-laxation.) Then place the dots on various items in your home or office to remind yourself to do a mini. Many people stick dots on the phone or computer, both of which can be a source of stress, or on the refrigerator if they tend to be "emotional eaters."

As with the relaxation response, the key to a successful mini is your breathing, so start with a few deep diaphragmatic breaths. Breathe through your nose, which helps to slow the pace of your breathing.

Chapter 4

Manage Your Stress

S TRESS CAN DAMAGE the heart by causing biochemical changes that constrict arteries and encourage the formation of blockages. If you have already suffered a heart attack or are at risk of developing heart disease, then stress will only exacerbate your medical condition. Even if you don't have many of the risk factors discussed in Chapter 2, stress alone can be toxic to your heart. You might not notice the damage caused by stress at first, but it wreaks havoc with your body over time.

Fortunately, you can learn to manage stress. In our Cardiac Wellness Program, we teach a stress management program based on two premises. First, most stress comes from the way we think or perceive events. Second, the thoughts that trigger stress are usually unrealistic and distorted. That means changing the way you think can greatly reduce your stress level.

This may seem impossible at first. But as with the relaxation response, you'll find that stress management is a skill that can be learned and gets easier with practice.

■ What Is Stress?

We all experience stress, but do we really know what stress is? Oddly enough, this common phenomenon has taken years to define. Ask an engineer about stress, and you'll learn about mechanical forces that can actually change the shape of a physical structure. Others, including some physicians, may define stress as the effect of external force, demand, or wear and tear on the body. Yet a third take, supported by research, indicates that much stress is a result of perceiving a threat to your well-being and feeling that you are unable to cope with that threat.

This is a subtle shift in emphasis, but an important one. It is your perception and appraisal of an event, rather than the event itself, that will determine whether you experience stress. This is actually good news. While you may not be able to change a particular situation, you can alter your perception of it and thus reduce your stress level.

Stress warning signs: Stress causes physical, emotional, behavioral, and even cognitive changes. Although stress warning signals vary from person to person, chances are that you will experience the same symptoms whenever you experience stress.

When you feel stress, you may have a knot in your stomach or your palms may sweat. Perhaps you snap at others or chew gum compulsively. You become easily rattled and upset. Or you may eat compulsively. Maybe you find it hard to think clearly and you completely lose your sense of humor. These are all signs that you are experiencing the stress response. Look at the list of typical stress warning signals in Table 4, page 92, and see which ones look familiar to you.

Stress Response: The stress response is more commonly known as the *fight-or-flight response*. As mentioned in Chapter 3, the fight-or-flight response evolved as a survival mechanism. It involves a

---

TABLE 4

STRESS WARNING SIGNALS

PHYSICAL SYMPTOMS

____ Headaches	____ Back pain
____ Indigestion	____ Tight neck, shoulders
____ Stomachaches	____ Racing heart
____ Sweaty palms	____ Restlessness
____ Sleep difficulties	____ Tiredness
____ Dizziness	____ Ringing in ears

BEHAVIORAL SYMPTOMS

____ Excessive smoking	____ Grinding of teeth
____ Bossiness	____ Overuse of alcohol
____ Compulsive gum chewing	____ Compulsive eating
____ Critical attitude toward others	____ Inability to get things done

EMOTIONAL SYMPTOMS

____ Crying	____ Overwhelming sense of
____ Nervousness, anxiety	pressure
____ Boredom—inability to find	____ Anger
meaning in things	____ Loneliness
____ Edginess—readiness to explode	____ Unhappiness for no
____ Feeling powerless to change things	reason
	____ Getting upset easily

COGNITIVE SYMPTOMS

____ Trouble thinking clearly	____ Inability to make decisions
____ Forgetfulness	____ Thoughts of running away
____ Lack of creativity	____ Constant worrying
____ Memory loss	____ Loss of sense of humor

---

powerful combination of physiologic responses that can help you survive a life-threatening situation.

The problem is, your brain doesn't distinguish between real-life threats and more routine types of stress, such as those caused by relationships, work, and family conflicts. Over time, chronic exposure to the physical changes caused by stress can contribute significantly to high blood pressure and heart disease.

TABLE 5

THE HOLMES SOCIAL READJUSTMENT RATING SCALE

Some events in life are more stressful than others. Although there are many tests and quizzes to measure stress, one of the most frequently cited is the Holmes Social Readjustment Rating Scale, which ranks forty-three life events according to degree of stress experienced by most people. Look at the list below and think about whether any of these events have happened to you in the last year. If so, expect them to have caused some degree of stress. Then think about events that stress you out in the course of a typical day. Are they on the list of top stressors? Or are you reacting to a minor problem as if it were a life-or-death situation?

Rank	Life Event	Stress Value
1	Death of spouse/life partner	100
2	Divorce	73
3	Marital separation	65
4	Detention in jail	63
5	Death of a close relative	63
6	Major personal illness or injury	53
7	Marriage	50
8	Getting fired	47
9	Marital reconciliation	45
10	Retirement	45
11	Change in family member's health	44
12	Pregnancy	40
13	Sexual problems	39
14	New baby	39
15	Business readjustment	39
16	Change in finances	38
17	Death of a good friend	37
18	Career change	36
19	Increase or decrease in number of arguments with spouse	35
20	Large mortgage or debt	31
21	Foreclosure of mortgage or loan	30
22	Change in job responsibilities	29

(continued on next page)

Rank	Life Event	Stress Value
23	Son or daughter leaves the "nest"	29
24	Conflict with in-laws	29
25	Outstanding personal achievement	28
26	Spouse stops working or begins new job	26
27	Beginning or end of school	26
28	Change in living conditions	25
29	Personal behavior change	25
30	Conflict with boss	23
31	Change in work hours or conditions	20
32	Move to new home	20
33	Change schools	20
34	Change in recreation	19
35	Change in church activities	19
36	Change in social activities	18
37	Low mortgage or debt	17
38	Change in sleeping habits	16
39	Change in number of family get-togethers	15
40	Change in eating habits	15
41	Vacation	13
42	Christmas	12
43	Minor traffic violation	11

To calculate your score, add the stress value for every listed event that has happened to you in the past year. If you score less than 150, you are least likely to experience a stress-related illness. If you score between 151 and 300 points, you are at significant risk. If you score 301 points or more, you are at greatest risk.

■ Common Myths about Stress

Before we go into more detail about the realities of stress, we'd like to examine some common myths.

Myth 1: All stress is bad. Actually, a little bit of stress can be quite good for you and it can enhance your thinking and performance.

There's even a law about this, named for Drs. Robert Yerkes and John Dodson of Harvard University, who first documented the relationship between stress and performance levels. Yerkes and Dodson conducted experiments showing that as stress levels increase, so does performance and efficiency—but only for so long. At a certain point, if stress continues to escalate, performance and efficiency will deteriorate. A task that involves too little challenge will bore you; one that applies too much pressure will make you feel overwhelmed and out of control. The key is to find a balance so that you are a top performer. As the psychologist Donald Tubesing once wrote, "Finding the right amount of stress is like adjusting the strings of a violin: too loose and you won't like the music; too tight and they might break."

Myth 2: I must feel stressed in order to succeed. This is a common myth among many of the patients in our Cardiac Wellness Program, who assume they must juggle multiple tasks and work all sorts of hours in order to succeed. In fact, research shows that taking things a little slower might make people more productive. Executives who establish priorities at work, delegate tasks, and leave their work behind them at the end of the day, it has been found, are more successful than colleagues who work all the time.

Myth 3: If I could just change my circumstances, I wouldn't feel as stressed as I do now. Much of the time, you will feel just as much stress in one situation as in another because your perception of an event—not the event itself—determines your stress level. Of course, some people and situations are toxic in themselves, and you are wise to avoid them. But before you make a drastic change, such as leaving a job or a relationship, think about how you can change your perception of a situation and your reaction to it. That may well be enough to reduce your stress level.

So much for the common myths: What about the realities of stress? Before you can manage your stress better, you first have to understand more about what causes it and how the stress response can escalate.

■ What Triggers Stress

A stress trigger is something that provokes a physiological stress response. Stress triggers can be external or internal.

Biogenic triggers: Coffee, tea, and amphetamines are examples of biogenic stressors—foods, drugs, and other substances that, after you ingest them, can trigger a stress response on their own. If you have ever had too much coffee on a particular morning and then experienced a rapid heartbeat or heart palpitations, you have experienced the strength of a physical stress response.

Psychosocial triggers: These triggers are much more significant than biogenic stressors when it comes to heart disease. Rather than the stress response being activated by an ingested compound, a psychosocial trigger involves interpreting an event in such a way that you feel threatened. This involves a one-two punch. First you perceive a threat to your well-being that seems overwhelming. Then you quickly (and subconsciously) appraise how well you can cope with the threat. If you feel you don't have appropriate resources to cope with a particular threat, you will feel stress.

There are three major types of psychosocial events that can serve as stress triggers. The first type is any major change that affects a large number of people. (A dramatic example of this type of trigger is the September 11, 2001, attacks on the United States.) Another trigger involves a major change that affects you and perhaps a few other people. Examples include loss of a job, a divorce, a car accident, and (on a more positive side) a promotion or the birth of a child. Finally, daily hassles also serve as stress triggers.

These include traffic jams, malfunctioning computer equipment, doctor's appointments, surprise assignments at work, and family squabbles. In comparing psychosocial triggers, research has concluded that the accumulation of daily "hassles" may be more harmful to your heart than major life changes.

■ How We Make Stress Worse

You are what you eat, as dietitians like to say. Here's another maxim: You are what you think. And for some, the way you think may only serve to exacerbate the effects of stress triggers.

We all experience life in a subjective manner. Two people walking down the same street, at the same time, will notice different things. That's because a constant stream of thoughts, wishes, and judgments—many of which we may not be conscious of—help us to perceive and interpret the world. These thoughts occur automatically and may seem to flow spontaneously, but they are really shaped by our underlying expectations and beliefs. It's as if we are all walking around with sunglasses that have different colored lenses. Some see a cheerful world through "rose-colored" glasses; others have a darker view of things.

Stop for a moment and try to remember the thoughts that were running through your head as you got dressed this morning. What were you saying to yourself? What were you thinking? Then think about how you felt.

Thoughts and moods are related. If you were thinking about a recent slight by a friend or a pressing deadline, then chances are you were feeling anxious, worried, maybe even angry as you got dressed. If you were thinking about something happy, such as an upcoming vacation or a visit with a friend, then chances are you felt upbeat and energized.

Happy or negative thoughts not only affect you emotionally; they have a physical effect as well. Negative thoughts can lead to headaches, low back pain, insomnia, and high blood pressure—all symptoms of stress. Negative thoughts can also result in changes in behavior, such as cigarette smoking, alcohol abuse, and overeating. None of this, of course, is good for your heart.

Although you will likely experience both positive and negative thoughts during the course of a typical day, it may surprise you to learn that many of your thoughts are distorted and unrealistic. Those lenses we mentioned earlier aren't only different colors, they also change the shape of what is out there—like 3D glasses. Or they have blinders that obscure your vision. And that warped perception of reality may be hurting your heart.

Remember that your mind does not know how to tell the difference between what is real and what is imagined. Imaging studies of the brain have shown that if someone actually looks at an object such as a house versus simply imagining that object, the same area in the brain lights up. That's why thinking about something scary will make you jumpy and thinking about something sad will make you cry. In the same way, constantly thinking about worst-case scenarios will make you tense.

Most of our automatic thoughts are negative. Theorists such as the psychologist Albert Ellis have shown these thoughts also tend to be knee-jerk reactions, based on irrational beliefs, rather than the result of careful analysis or insightful thinking. Have you ever encountered a situation where you immediately assumed the worst—and then it didn't turn out as badly as you thought it would? That's an example of automatic thinking. Such thoughts usually come on quickly; you may not even be conscious that you are thinking. The problem is, you may take this automatic thought—your perception—as reality. And after a while, if we think something often enough, we begin to believe it.

Try to recognize automatic thoughts as they occur to you. Then analyze the situation and the automatic thought it provokes. Does your thinking contain one or more of the characteristics listed in Sidebar 14, page 99? If so, you may be suffering from what the psychologist and author David D. Burns has called "cognitive

---

AUTOMATIC THOUGHTS

Automatic thoughts are easy to identify once you know what to watch for. The following words are usually red flags for negative automatic thoughts:

- Always
- Must
- Never
- Ought
- Should

Automatic thoughts sound like this:

- "Oh no!"
- "Why me?"
- "I can't stand this!"
- "I'm not good enough!"
- "Nothing will ever change."
- "This always happens to me."
- "I'll never get everything done."
- "How can I be so stupid?"
- "I should have done better."
- "Things will never change."

---

distortions." Burns identified ten broad types of cognitive distortions; we've added a few of our own based on the work of Ellis and Greiger.

All or nothing: Situations are perceived as one way or the other. Everything is black or white; nothing is ever gray. If you make a mistake, you declare yourself a total failure. For example, you quit smoking for three months but then have one cigarette at a party; you decide you'll never succeed at quitting and take up smoking again.

Generalization: When you experience a single negative event, you see it as part of a lifelong continuum. For instance, if you find yourself standing in the slowest-moving line in a grocery store, you think, "I always pick the wrong line." If your spouse is late for dinner and forgets to call to let you know, you think things like, "he always does this to me." If you are passed over for a promotion at work, you conclude that you will never get ahead in your career.

Mental filter: You focus so much on the negative aspect of a situation that you fail to see anything positive in it. It's as if you are filtering out all the light and only see darkness. For instance, during your annual job review your boss has mostly praise for your performance but asks if you could work on your temper and not be so short with people. You fixate on the criticism and soon become convinced your boss hates you and you might be fired. Another example: You're at a party, having a good time, when a friend asks if you've gained a little weight recently. Your evening is ruined.

Disqualifying the positive: When someone pays you a compliment, you dismiss or devalue it. You don't respond by saying thank you. Instead you say, "Anyone could have done it." Or you think to yourself, "They're just being nice." Although you might think you're being modest by deflecting praise, this type of cognitive distortion eventually makes you blind to anything positive in life. It's a way of turning positive events into negative ones.

Jumping to conclusions: This is the tendency to predict the future or what someone is thinking without ever evaluating the facts of a situation. There are two common variations of this distortion.

Mind reading: You make assumptions about what someone else is thinking without verifying it. For example, after giving a presentation at a business meeting, you ask for questions and there are none. You assume everyone hated the presentation and can't wait to get out of the room. Or your spouse tells you, "The children understand that we have to tighten our belts until you feel good enough to return to work full time." You think, "They think I'm a failure."

Fortune telling: Before you do something, you anticipate a negative outcome. In some cases, you don't even try to act because you are convinced you will fail. For example, you decide not to ask your boss if you can work from home two days a week, because you *know* she'll say no, so what's the point. If you have a heart attack, you declare that you'll never be well again.

Magnification: You blow a negative event out of proportion, so that even a minor occurrence becomes a catastrophe. For instance, it rains on the morning of your daughter's wedding, and you conclude that nothing else that day is going to go right and guests will have a lousy time. The result: You may be in a foul mood on what should be one of the happiest days of your life. Or you find out that your refrigerator must be replaced, and you think, "That's it, I guess we're not going on vacation this year since all our money is going to go toward home repairs."

Minimalization: This is the exact opposite of magnification. You tend to dismiss or belittle the importance of anything good that happens. For instance, you receive a raise at work but you think, "What's the use? Uncle Sam will take half the money and what's left doesn't amount to much." Or someone compliments you on your green thumb, and you say, "It's no big deal."

Emotional reasoning: You think that whatever you are feeling is an accurate indicator of your identity and self-worth. Your mood defines who you are. For instance, if you feel anxious, you think, "It's because I'm no good at anything." Or if you feel jealous, you think, "It's because I'm not as good as other people and never will be."

Should statements: You often find yourself saying or thinking "I should do this" or "I must do that." The result is that you may feel inadequate, pressured, anxious, resentful, and completely unmotivated. "Should" statements may bring to mind an image of an overbearing parent or teacher wagging a finger at you. Albert Ellis called should statements a form of "musterbation."

Labeling and mislabeling: You define yourself, other people, and situations simplistically, on the basis of one negative event, rather than seeing complexity and variation. For instance, you skip your daily walk because you're tired, and then you think, "I'm such a lazy slob." Or you make a mistake, and you think, "I'm such a loser." You have a bad day at work, and you think, "This job stinks." If you perform poorly on a particular task you conclude that you are a total failure.

Personalization: Somehow everything is your fault, even if you have nothing to do with it. For instance, your child does not play well at a softball game, and you think, "It's all my fault. I'm a lousy parent. I didn't spend enough time practicing ball with my child." Or one of your employees doesn't complete a task on time, and you think, "I should have motivated him better."

Perfectionism: No matter how well you do something, it is never good enough unless it is perfect. You hold similarly high expectations for other people. When, for instance, you score 95 on a test, you are disappointed because it wasn't 100. You make a minor mistake and think, "I will never get it right."

Approval seeking: You must have the constant approval of all the significant people in your life. If they don't express that approval at all times, you feel awful. For example, you handle a particularly difficult customer at work, but your boss doesn't give you the pat on the back you were expecting. Or you go to great trouble to cook a special dinner one night, but your spouse doesn't even seem to notice.

Self-righteous: People should always act the way *you* think is right; if they don't, they're wrong and should be punished. For instance, you're at a business event and one of your colleagues decides to have a glass of wine rather than the seltzer water that you are drinking; you're outraged, and if you were the boss, you'd demote that person. Or you notice that your neighbor's children are outside after eight o'clock at night, while yours are safely inside,

THE DENTIST'S APPOINTMENT

A patient we'll call Sheila was eager to talk about her most recent stressful experience. She was laughing now that it was over, but she hadn't been laughing at the time it happened. We've added italicized descriptions of the type of automatic thoughts she is demonstrating.

Sheila's story: "My husband had an appointment for a root canal," she said, "and I said I'd drive him there and then do some shopping at the mall instead of waiting in the dentist's office." The appointment was for 2 P.M. in a town about twenty minutes away. By 1:30, she was calling up the stairs impatiently: "Ralph, you're going to be late! Hurry up!" It took Ralph another five minutes to get ready, but at last he came downstairs and the two of them headed out the door.

They began bickering in the car. "We've got plenty of time," Ralph said.

"What if there's traffic?" Sheila pointed out. And recounting the story to the class at the Cardiac Wellness Program, she added, "He always does this. Always *(generalization)*. He's the kind of person who wants everyone else to do his worrying for him."

As they drove, Sheila fumed silently. "We'll never get there," she thought to herself *(fortune telling)*. "Why did I even agree to do this? I should have let him drive himself!" *(should statement)*.

They pulled in to the office five minutes before the appointment, and Sheila began to relax when she saw the door close behind Ralph. She dabbed her face with powder and got ready to back out of the parking lot, when the dentist's door opened—and there was Ralph. He climbed back into the car.

"He's in his other office today," Ralph said, "the next town over."

Sheila was so furious she could barely speak. She could feel her face flushing and she started to sweat. Ralph, meanwhile, looked completely relaxed. She told the class: "It's always like this. He couldn't care less, and I'm the one who's having a heart attack" *(jumping to conclusions; generalization)*.

MONIQUE'S STORY

Read the following story. Can you identify some of Monique's cognitive distortions? (Answers below.)

A patient we'll call Monique is a gourmet cook who loves to entertain. One week she arrived at the Cardiac Wellness Program enthusiastic about a party she and her husband would be hosting that weekend. Good weather was predicted, and Monique looked forward to getting everything ready.

At the next week's class, we asked her how the party had gone. "Oh, it was awful!" she said, clearly depressed.

Other members of the class, concerned, asked her what had gone wrong. "Didn't people enjoy themselves?"

"They had a good time," Monique said.

"Was there some glitch with the tent?"

"No, the tent was up the day before and people seemed to enjoy the shade."

"Wasn't the food good?"

"Everything was great," Monique said, "until I tasted the dill potato salad and realized I'd added too much dill to it." For Monique, the whole party had been ruined *(cognitive distortions: magnification, perfectionism; all or nothing; mental filter)*.

---

and decide that your neighbors are bad parents and you're not sure you want your children playing with theirs any longer.

■ The Stress Cycle

As we encounter stress throughout the day, our negative automatic thoughts fuel a negative stress cycle, which can take on a life of its own. Here's how it works: We encounter something

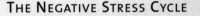

TABLE 6

THE NEGATIVE STRESS CYCLE

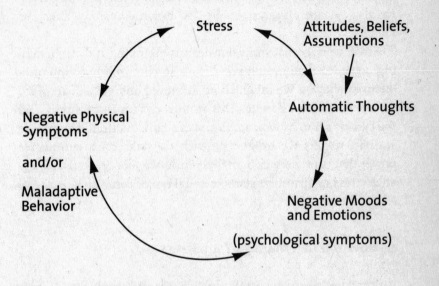

Your doctor's appointment is at 11 A.M.
It's now 11:15, and you have no idea how long you'll have to wait,
which starts the cycle.

Breath is shallow and rapid.   "This always happens to me."
Palms are sweaty.   "Now I'll miss my lunch date."
Heart is pounding.   "Doctors are always so inconsiderate of
                                      other people's time."
                                      "I'll never be seen."
                                      "No wonder I have high blood pressure."

Anger
Frustration
Feeling victimized

The negative stress cycle builds on itself. Frank, whose story is summarized above, started experiencing stress at 11:15 A.M., when he realized the doctor was running late. By 11:30 the doctor was ready to see him, but Frank was shaking and having trouble breathing. Frank's initial stress reactions were compounded by his thinking and emotions.

stressful, which not only activates the fight-or-flight response but also triggers negative automatic thoughts. The negative thoughts are like gasoline being poured on a fire—they heighten our stress response. So, as our muscles tense and our blood pressure rises, we also "steam up" emotionally and become anxious, angry, or hostile.

Small wonder that while our heart is pounding and our breathing becomes shallow and rapid, we also succumb to counterproductive behavior. We might shout at a loved one, eat a quart of ice cream, or grab a cigarette. This in turn creates more stress, and the cycle is set in motion again and can build on itself. Soon those stressful events we experience each day take on a cumulative power that is far greater than their sum. We literally feed the negative stress cycle until it starts to spiral out of control.

■ How You Can Manage Your Stress

We can't promise you a stress-free life. No one can do that. But we can offer some guidance on how to better manage your stress.

Think about fire control for a moment. Putting out a brushfire is a lot easier than fighting a full-blown forest fire. Our stress management advice works along the same lines. We don't promise to eliminate stress from your life, but we can provide you with techniques to help you recognize and change the way you perceive and react to an event, so that a minor annoyance doesn't escalate into an overwhelming situation.

■ Recognize the Early Warning Signals

Before you can manage stress, you first have to realize that you are experiencing it. Sadly, most of us carry around so much residual tension that we can become less sensitized to it. We might think our tense state normal.

One way to detect stress would be to walk around with a blood pressure monitor. This way you could literally see your blood pressure increase. Or you could have someone monitor your heart rate. Of course, neither approach is practical.

■ Stress Awareness Exercise

The best approach is to learn to recognize your stress warning signs. Over the next week, pay attention whenever you feel stress. Identify what events or situations trigger the stress response and what stress warning signals you notice. (You may want to take another look at the list of stress warning signals in Table 4, page 92, to familiarize yourself with them.) It's important to write this information down as soon as possible so that you won't forget it.

TABLE 7
STRESS AWARENESS LOG

Time	Stressful Event	Physical and Emotional Feelings
____	_____	_____
____	_____	_____
____	_____	_____
____	_____	_____
____	_____	_____

■ Change the Way You Think

As we mentioned earlier in this chapter, negative automatic thoughts only exacerbate the stress response. Fortunately, you can change your thought processes by using a therapeutic technique known as *cognitive restructuring*—changing the way you think and perceive a given event. This may seem impossible, but in fact you can learn new mind postures pretty much the same way that you learn a new body posture.

Let's say, for instance, that you develop tingling in your hands and arms while working at a computer. After consulting an ergonomics manual, you might readjust the height of your chair and position your arms at a 90-degree angle to the keyboard in order to relieve stress on your hands and wrists.

You use much the same approach with cognitive restructuring. First you identify thoughts and beliefs that are irrational and self-defeating. Then you learn about new ways of thinking and practice them, and soon they become second nature.

To make the process easier, we've broken it down into four steps: stop, breathe, reflect, and choose.

Step 1: Stop: The next time you start feeling stress, simply say *stop* to yourself. The key here is to say the word. This literally stops the negative stress cycle in its tracks.

Step 2: Breathe: After you say stop, breathe deeply from your diaphragm. Repeat this a few times. It reduces physical tension and helps you relax. This in turn will help reduce your anxiety and worry levels so that you can think more clearly.

Step 3: Reflect: Once you have stopped the cycle, you can focus your energy on the problem at hand and appraise the situation. First, identify the stressful situation and your physical and emotional stress warning signs using columns 1 and 2 in the cognitive restructuring log (Table 8, pages 110 to 113). Write down your automatic thoughts in column 3. What cognitive distortions do your automatic thoughts contain? Write those down in column 4.

Step 4: Choose: Now that you're aware of how your thinking can become distorted, the next step is to challenge the distortion and readjust your view of reality. Dr. Ellis, the psychologist we mentioned earlier in this chapter, developed a model known as *rational emotive therapy* to do just that. The point is to ask yourself: How else can I think about the situation? What else can I do? Try it, even if at first you don't trust the alternative view.

For instance, let's say you are prone to catastrophic thinking. Your car blows a tire and as you call AAA, you think, "Now I bet the whole car is going to fall apart, and I'll end up paying thousands of dollars in repairs and will never get rid of my credit card debt." Challenge the catastrophe. Try thinking, "Oh well, I'll have to replace the tire and that's going to set me back a hundred dollars." Or how about, "Gee, I'm glad the tire blew on this side street while I was driving slowly. It would have been much worse if I were on the highway."

Now identify some alternative responses to your own situation. Literally challenge the negative impulse and try to see a situation differently, in a more positive light. For instance, I can handle this, it's one step at a time, I'm doing the best I can, I'll get through this. Write your responses in column 5. Now think about how you feel since you've identified new options. Write that in column 6.

Changing the way you think will take time and practice, much like learning a new dance step. At first it will feel awkward to go against the grain of who you are, but with time it will become easier. Use the cognitive restructuring log to help you learn the process. It's the easiest and fastest way to become aware of how your thoughts affect your emotions. Then you can literally think on paper about alternatives, and afterward decide on a new course of action. Writing it down makes it real.

TABLE 8

COGNITIVE RESTRUCTURING LOG

Keep track of events that make you feel stress and then try to analyze what happened, using the following grid to help you better manage the event in the future. Try keeping the log for a couple of weeks. We've included a sample response from a patient in the Cardiac Wellness Program, and left lines blank so that you can record your own thoughts and experiences.

Stressful Event *Briefly describe what happened.*	Stress Warning Signals *Identify your physical signs and feelings.*	Automatic Thoughts *What were your immediate thoughts?*	Cognitive Distortions *Identify the distortions (see pages 99 to 102).*	Rational Response *How else might you think about the situation and what might you do to cope?*	Outcome *How do you feel now?*
Policeman gave me a speeding ticket.	Palms sweat so much my hands slipped off the steering wheel. Felt flushed. I couldn't breathe and my voice was raspy as I tried to explain why I shouldn't get the ticket.	This always happens to me, whereas other people get away with it. Why now? I'm already late for my meeting. My whole day is ruined	Generalization (Do you *really* always get speeding tickets?) Awfulizing and fortune telling (My whole day is ruined.)	It's just a speeding ticket. I can handle this. It's just a bump in the road. I'm sure my wife will understand. The cops are just enforcing the rules.	Calm. Feel less like a victim and more in control.

Stuck in traffic	Blew the horn out of frustration. Squirmed in the seat and tried to see around the cars to see what the problem was. Started muttering, "Come on, come on, let's get the show on the road."	How am I going to explain this to my wife? She is going to be so upset. She'll never understand. She'll think I'm a reckless driver. The cops should be looking for "real" criminals. There are too many morons on the roads. Nobody knows how to drive. Where are the cops when you need them? They should be trying to solve this tie-up? I'm never going to make it to my appointment.	Jumping to conclusions, fortune telling. (Your wife will be angry and will conclude you're reckless.) Self-righteous (The cops should be enforcing the laws *you* consider important.) Generalization and labeling (All the other drivers are incompetent.) Should statements (The cops *should* be solving this.) All-or-nothing thinking, fortune telling, and magnification (I'll never make it to the appointment.)	It's just a delay. The traffic will clear up eventually. Next time I'll allow more time so that this doesn't happen again. Maybe I should listen to some music or do a "mini"; it will get my mind off things.	Peaceful Enjoying some time alone before the day's demands begin.

(continued)

Stressful Event *Briefly describe what happened.*	Stress Warning Signals *Identify your physical signs and feelings.*	Automatic Thoughts *What were your immediate thoughts?*	Cognitive Distortions *Identify the distortions (see pages 99 to 102).*	Rational Response *How else might you think about the situation and what else might you do to cope?*	Outcome *How do you feel now?*
Stuck in traffic *(cont.)*	When a car in another lane tried to cut in front of me, I wouldn't let it. Heart pounding in chest.	Who does that other driver think I am, some little patsy who will let him get in front of me? What if the car starts to overheat?	Mind reading (The other driver thinks you're a patsy.) Awfulizing and fortune telling (The car may overheat.)	I'll reach my destination eventually. I'll let that guy cut in front of me. Why not? We're not moving very fast anyway.	
Waiting in a doctor's office	Angry, hurt	This always happens to me. He is so rude, making me wait. He doesn't care about me.	Generalization Labeling Magnification	I can wait. I have a book I can read. He may have an emergency with another patient.	Calm Feel less like a put-upon patient and more like a partner in care.

No wonder I have high blood pressure.	Jumping to conclusions	I'll do the best that I can.	
This is a waste of my time.	Awfulizing	I'll probably only be a few minutes late for work.	
I'll never get to work.	Fortune telling		
Write about your own stressful events and reactions in these spaces.			

JOAN'S STORY

Identify Joan's stress warning signals and cognitive distortions based on the story below. Then think about stressful events in your own life. Can you analyze what happened and what cognitive distortions might have affected your own thinking and reactions?

When a patient we'll call Joan began participating in the Cardiac Wellness Program, she suffered from high blood pressure, elevated cholesterol levels, and angina. Yet to look at her, she was the picture of health: Her weight was well within the normal range and she was busy and active. At fifty-five, she had few apparent risk factors for heart disease. But during our sessions on stress management, it became clear why she had entered the program.

The previous Saturday, her eighteen-year-old son had promised to be home by 1 A.M. Though Joan didn't intend to stay up and wait for him, she couldn't sleep because she kept checking the clock. Then she would toss and turn and check the clock again. By 1:30 A.M. she had become frantic. "I knew I shouldn't have given him my car. I just knew he'd been in a car accident," Joan told the other Cardiac Wellness Program participants. "All of a sudden, my heart started pounding and I couldn't breathe. I thought, he's probably dead! I tried to call the police, but my hands were shaking so badly I couldn't dial the phone."

Just then, a car pulled in to the driveway: her son, safe and sound. It turns out he'd lost track of the time. But Joan still could not relax. "I was up half the night, long after he'd fallen asleep. I just couldn't settle down. Kids are so irresponsible these days. No wonder I have heart problems. I will never survive these teenage years! It's downhill from here."

Stress Warning Signals

____ Tossing and turning in bed
____ Heart pounding
____ Trouble breathing

Cognitive Symptoms	Examples
____ Jumping to conclusions	"I just knew he'd been in a car accident."
____ Awfulizing	"He's probably dead." "It's downhill from here."
____ All-or-nothing thinking	"Kids are so irresponsible these days."
____ Fortune telling	"I will never survive these teenage years!"

In class, we encouraged Joan to challenge her automatic thoughts. Instead of jumping to conclusions, in the future she could consider alternative explanations for why her son was late. After all, teenagers tend to lose track of time, especially when they're with friends. Or he might have had a flat tire and was trying to fix it. Even if her son had been in a car accident, it could have been a minor fender bender and not a catastrophe. Joan agreed that these were all more likely than the deadly accident she'd envisioned. Finally, we offered practical suggestions to help her avoid this situation in the future, such as giving her son a cell phone so that she could reach him if she was worried.

___

Sidebar 18

The Goose-in-a-Bottle Exercise

Try this exercise designed to challenge negative thoughts. Our patients enjoy it.

Imagine that there is a large, wide-bottomed glass vase with a very plump and happy goose inside (see illustration on page 116). Now think about how you will get the goose out of the vase without either

breaking the glass or hurting the goose. Think carefully. It may help
to consider how a full-grown goose got itself stuck in the vase in the
first place.

The answer? It's impossible for a goose to become wedged into a
glass vase. You imagined him there! And you can imagine him out of
it. Yet all too often we spend time, energy, and pain worrying about
something that exists only in our imagination.

A patient we'll call Jane left her office and got into her car to drive
home one day. As she drove, she remembered that she had asked her
husband to defrost some chicken that morning so that they could eat
it for dinner. "He always forgets to do things like that," Jane thought
to herself. "He really doesn't do his fair share of chores, come to
think of it." One thought led to another. Soon Jane was imagining the
fight they would have when she got home: what she would say, how

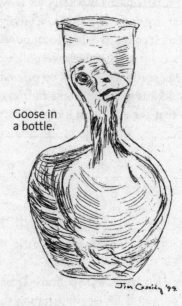

Goose in
a bottle.

Figure 19: Goose in a bottle

he would respond, the shouting argument, the trial separation, the divorce, how tough it would be to be single again, and so on. By the time she got home, she was completely worn out and emotionally depleted. So imagine her surprise when she walked in the door to find that her husband had not only defrosted the chicken, he'd put it in the oven to bake!

When you find yourself worrying about something, challenge yourself. Is the problem real—or the equivalent of a goose in a bottle?

CHANGING THE FAMILY STRESS DYNAMIC

A man we'll call John was a patient in our Cardiac Wellness Program. He and his wife, Ellen, raised three children, who were now married. John and Ellen were just getting used to having an "empty nest" again when John suffered a heart attack. It proved to be a frightening and life-changing event for both of them. Do you recognize in yourself or your loved one any of the stress reactions and cognitive distortions that follow in their story? If so, pay attention to how John and Ellen learned to think differently about their situation and reduce their stress levels.

John's story: "This heart attack hit me out of the blue. Sure, I'd put on a few pounds over the years, and my wife had been after me for years to quit smoking, but I never really thought it would happen to me. I don't remember the first days at the hospital very well; I must have been in a daze. The hardest part actually began when they sent me home. Maybe I had too much time to think. I'd sit there thinking, 'Why me? I should have taken better care of myself. I should have seen this coming *(should statements)*. This is all my fault *(personalization)*. I'm such a jerk for not being able to quit smoking before this' *(labeling)*.

"My kids came to see me, to cheer me up, but somehow that made it worse. I thought, 'I've let my family down *(jumping to conclusions)*. I'll never get to see my grandchildren grow up' *(fortune telling, magnification)*. Ellen tried too, but the more she encouraged me the more depressed I felt. We went for a walk one night, because the doctor told me to get some exercise, and I couldn't keep up with her. I just didn't have the energy. I got really discouraged and thought, 'I'll never get better *(generalization, fortune telling)*. If I can't even walk, I'll never be able to play golf or do other things I always enjoyed *(jumping to conclusions)*. It's all downhill from here' " *(magnification)*.

Ellen's reaction: "Once I got over the initial shock, I was angry— at John, at myself, at the world. You know, he was always skipping lunch and eating junk food out of the vending machine *(generalization)*. His work was too pressured, that was the problem; he should have changed jobs. And he should have listened to me when I told him to eat better food and to slow down *(should statements)*. It's his fault that this happened! *(blame)*.

Then I started to worry. I couldn't sleep at night; I found myself listening to his breathing to make sure he was all right. I thought, 'What if he can't return to work? We'll have to sell the house *(jumping to conclusions, fortune telling)*. Life will never be the same for us. We'll always feel as though we are walking on eggshells, waiting for something else to happen' " *(fortune telling)*.

John and Ellen both took time to fill out the cognitive restructuring log to help challenge their distorted thinking and adopt a more positive and productive attitude. Not surprisingly, their stress levels also dropped. Although there are no guarantees that John will not get sick again, the couple is trying to remain optimistic and cope better with their new reality. Here are some of the rational responses John and Ellen developed after completing the cognitive restructuring log:

John's Restructured Thoughts	Ellen's Restructured Thoughts
I am disappointed that I have heart disease.	I am really frightened. It's not all his fault.
I could have taken better care of myself, but I did quit smoking.	He did quit smoking; that was a big step.

I really have been trying to eat better.

I can handle this.

I'll take it one step at a time.

If I take better care of myself, I should be able to live a normal life.

I plan on being around to see my grandchildren grow up.

It's really not all my fault. I have a family history of heart disease. Some of this is genetic.

The doctor said I should be able to do anything in moderation. He actually encouraged me to be active.

We could both eat better but overall we try to eat healthfully.

The doctor said he will be okay.

I'm not going to blow this out of proportion.

It's one day at a time.

I'm sure he can go back to work.

We both could learn to manage stress better.

Maybe we could join a class together.

It may be difficult at first, but I know that we can get through this together.

■ Communicate Better

Much of what we've discussed so far involves making internal changes in the way you (and perhaps your loved ones) think and perceive experience. But another aspect of stress management involves external changes in the way you communicate with others.

Communication involves the exchange of information between individuals. That exchange can be verbal, which involves both what you say and how you say it. It can also take the form of written expression such as a letter or an E-mail.

Another aspect of communication is the way you listen to other people and how well you understand them. This involves not only hearing words but also putting yourself in another person's "shoes" to understand his or her perception of a situation.

Finally, communication can be nonverbal. Your body language, facial expressions, eye contact, gestures, and actions may all convey as much or more information than your words.

Learning how to communicate more effectively is important for heart health because it helps you to manage stress better. It also enhances your sense of self-esteem, providing you with a hardy internal buffer, and improves your relationships with others. If you do not communicate effectively, you are likely to become angry and hostile—and that only harms your heart.

■ Four Communication Styles

There are four basic ways that people communicate: aggressive, assertive, passive, and passive-aggressive. Only one of these styles is productive. In the brief descriptions below, think of how you would communicate in a difficult situation. For instance, let's suppose you had a hard day at work and are tired. You've promised your spouse that you'll pick up a few things at the grocery store on the way home. So you race through the store, tossing bread and milk and a few other items into your cart, and then make a beeline for the express checkout line, the one with the sign that says "ten items or fewer." And there, standing right in front of you, is someone with at least fifteen items. Which of the following statements describes how you would probably react?

Option 1: You would poke the person on the shoulder and say, "Hey, what do you think you're doing? This is the express lane. You have too many items. Go over to that other line!"

Option 2: You would tap the person on the shoulder and say, "Excuse me, you may not realize that this is an express lane for people with fewer than ten items. Please go to another line."

Option 3: You want to say something in your own defense, but you don't. You just stand there and awfulize the situation, and think:

"People are so irresponsible. I'll never get home. This always happens to me."

Option 4: You tap your foot and exhale loudly with disgust. Maybe you even bump into the offending person.

Now see what each option reveals about your communication style.

Style 1—Aggressive: Someone who communicates aggressively believes, "I count, but you don't." Aggressive communicators always seem to be on the attack. The language they use is threatening and often hostile. This only serves to escalate emotions, turning a minor situation into a conflict.

Style 2—Assertive: People who are assertive believe, "I count and you count." This shows in their communication, as they strike a balanced tone. The language they use is not emotional. It acknowledges the other person's perspective, but also allows their own opinion to be heard.

Style 3—Passive: Passive communicators tend to think, "You count, but I don't." So they do and say nothing, even in a situation that bothers them.

Style 4—Passive-Aggressive: People who communicate in this way think, "I count, but I won't let you know it directly." Of all the communication styles this may be the least productive, because it leaves the other person guessing why you are (or are not) doing something or why you seem angry.

Assertive communication is best. It enables you to express your feelings, opinions, and positions in a way that is honest and also respectful of another person. It is a style that allows room for negotiation and choice. If you want to become more assertive in your communications, you can. But it takes work and practice.

■ The Four A's of Assertive Communication

You can change your communication style. Let's say, for instance, that you have spent hours working on a report for your boss. Then he shows up in your office and says, "You did a lousy job on this report." An aggressive person might reply, "What do you expect? You didn't give me enough time." A passive person might accept the report silently and sit there just seething for the next hour. A passive-aggressive person might sit silently for a few moments, then slam the door loudly when the boss leaves the room.

Now consider how to handle the same situation by communicating assertively, using this four-step process.

Acknowledge: Start by acknowledging in some way that you hear and understand the other person's position. This will prevent a situation from becoming overly emotional and opens the door for negotiation. To follow with the example above, say something like, "I'm sorry you feel that I did such a lousy job with that report." This indicates that you have heard what your boss was saying— even if you don't agree with it.

Ask for more: If you feel defensive or put upon, you may be jumping to conclusions about the other person's viewpoint. Try asking for more information, which both buys you time to calm down and helps you to better understand what the person is saying. You might say to your boss, "I would really like to talk to you some more about this, and find out which sections need to be improved."

Align with the positive: Identify the common goals you share with another person. Focus on the task, not the boss—or yourself. Say something like, "I really want to make this report as great as possible."

Add your own: Now that you've defused the situation and focused attention back on the central issue, it's time to assert your own opinions, viewpoints, and needs. Say, for instance, "Could we discuss this now or set up an appointment to talk? That way I'll better understand your expectations as I rewrite the report."

Sometimes all four steps can be telescoped into a few brief sentences. Let's say, for example, you have that hard day and then get stuck in a long line at the grocery store. By the time you get home, you are frustrated and looking for some comfort. But when you open the door your spouse says, "What took you so long? We've got to get dinner started so that we can get to the parent-teacher conference tonight." What do you do?

An aggressive person might shout: "All you ever do is nag. I don't need any more aggravation today." A passive person might say nothing but develop a splitting headache and remain sullen for the rest of the evening. A passive-aggressive person might slam the bag of groceries down on the counter and stomp off into the bedroom.

An assertive person will say something like: "I had a really bad day today. Right now, I just need someone to listen to me for a few minutes. We can still make it to the parent-teacher conference on time."

■ Learn to Listen Better

Listening productively is an art and a skill. It takes more than just hearing spoken words. A productive listener displays empathy: He appreciates another person's reality without making a judgment. So often when we listen we do just the opposite: We formulate responses and advice even before the other person is finished speaking.

To achieve empathy, do three things. First, listen in an active and nonjudgmental way. Second, be sensitive to the other person's feelings, which may not be expressed in words. Third, communicate your understanding of what is being said to you, verbally and nonverbally, to the person who is speaking.

To get better at listening, try the empathy exercise in Sidebar 20, page 125. Listening with empathy will improve your communication skills and enable you to connect better with other people. That in turn will reduce your stress level.

■ Learn from Stress-Hardy People

Our work builds on research that has shown some people are more stress-resistant than others. When psychologist Suzanne Kobasa of the University of Chicago conducted research in this area, she found that people who were most resistant to stress shared three key characteristics, all beginning with the letter C.

They feel in **control** of their life, knowing they could make choices that would influence the outcome of events. They enjoy **challenges**, which they view as opportunities rather than threats. Finally, they are **committed** to (rather than alienated from) their work, family, and home life. In her studies, Kobasa found that such "stress hardy" people are less likely than others to become ill or be absent from work. To these three "C's," we have added a fourth: **closeness.** We've found, by working with patients and through our research, that personal relationships and other types of social support can provide a powerful buffer against stress (more on this in Chapter 5).

Another approach to stress hardiness is offered by Dr. Barrie Greiff, a psychiatrist and business consultant who is also a former professor at Harvard Business School. Greiff has identified what he terms the "five L's of success," personal habits correlated with health and happiness. People willing to engage in the five L's on a regular basis also tend to embrace life fully rather than hide from it.

EMPATHY EXERCISE

- Find a partner. Although you can choose a friend or someone you work with, this exercise is particularly beneficial if you work with your spouse, significant other, or child, as it may help to improve understanding—and thus communication—between you.
- Talk for five minutes about a stressful situation and how you handled it. Try to talk only about the facts of the situation, not the emotions it caused.
- Your partner should pay attention to the facts, but also try to discern your emotions from your words, body language, and facial expressions.
- Once you stop speaking, both you and your partner should silently, and on separate slips of paper, list the emotions you experienced based on this event.
- Compare lists. How well did your partner guess which emotions you were feeling?
- Now switch roles. As your partner speaks, try to quiet your own inner voice so that you can listen to his or her experience. Compare notes again.

After the exercise, ask yourselves these questions:

Was it difficult to listen? Did you find you wanted to interrupt your partner to offer advice? Were you thinking about how you would have handled the situation differently? Or were you able to empathize with your partner—did the emotions you detected match the ones he or she felt?

From the perspective of the person talking, did you feel that you were heard? How did that feel?

Learn: People willing to learn also tend to welcome new experiences rather than resist or worry about them.

Labor: People who work at something that they find satisfying and meaningful tend to be more positive than those who slog away at a job they despise.

Love: People who are in loving and reciprocal relationships with spouses, partners, or even friends develop an inner strength that helps them be more positive.

Laugh: A sense of humor in response to a situation, being able to laugh at oneself or with others, helps people to view life in a more positive way.

Let go: People who are able to recognize times when they are not in control of something and let go mentally have more energy to direct during situations in which they do have control.

■ Some Final Thoughts about Stress Management

The techniques described in this chapter should help you to create stress buffers that will reduce the toxic effects of stress on your heart and the rest of your body. Final pieces of advice include:

Use "I" messages: "I" messages convey your present emotions without blaming another person for causing those emotions. They sound less like attacks and more like explanations. "I" messages have a three-part structure and always begin with *I* (hence the name). For example, "I was frustrated when you forgot to take out the trash because I thought we agreed you would do that for me." Blame statements, on the other hand, often begin with the word *you* and tend to sound like accusations. For example: "You forgot to take out the trash again!"

Try to reframe blame statements into "I" statements using the grid we've provided.

Just say no: If you are feeling stress because you have taken on too many obligations, outside activities, or are responding to unreasonable demands on your time, you do have an option: Say no. Don't take unrewarding activities on in the first place. If you find yourself already "stuck" in a situation, then try to extricate yourself. If you feel guilty when you say no, then begin by saying no to small things. Chances are you will get better at it and gain the confidence to say no to big things as well.

TABLE 9

CONSTRUCTING "I" STATEMENTS

I FEEL (FILL IN EMOTION)	WHEN YOU (FILL IN BEHAVIOR)	BECAUSE (FILL IN EXPLANATION)
I was concerned _____	when you said _____	because I thought that _____

Here's how some of our patients filled this in:

I was worried	*when you were late and didn't call me*	*because I thought you'd been in a car accident.*
I was upset	*when you called on me in the meeting*	*because I would have responded better if you'd given me some time to prepare.*

Now try it yourself:

I was _____	when you _____	because I _____.
I was _____	when you _____	because I _____.
I was _____	when you _____	because I _____.
I was _____	when you _____	because I _____.

Ask directly for what you want: Don't assume that people will understand what you want or need from them. Sometimes you have to make it clear to them—even if they are close friends or family members. Don't be afraid to ask for what you want. Let's say that you come home from work and your spouse immediately starts ranting about his or her own bad day. Try saying something like: "I really want to listen to what you have to say, but I just need five minutes to get into more comfortable clothes and unwind a little. Then maybe we can make some tea and talk in the living room." Or: "I would like to help you but right now my plate is too full."

Go easy on yourself: As you try to put our advice into practice, don't stress out as you try to become unstressed. Change is an ongoing process and takes time. Congratulate yourself for even trying, and make each step count.

Chapter 5

Dealing with Emotions

Heartfelt. Heartsick. Heartthrob. Heartache. The connection between heart and emotion is not only embedded in everyday words and phrases, but has also been recognized in classic literature and texts. "A cheerful heart is good medicine," according to the seventeenth Proverb in the Bible. "A light heart lives long," proclaims Katherine in William Shakespeare's play *Love's Labor's Lost*. As discussed in Chapter 2, a substantial body of research has convinced many of us in the medical community that we need to take emotions seriously, especially when it comes to heart disease.

In this chapter, we'll focus more on the solution than the problem, providing information and exercises that will help you heal or open your heart. Patients in our Cardiac Wellness Program find that the classes on emotional healing are the most difficult in the thirteen-week series—and also the most helpful. For good reason: Acknowledging emotions and seeking out sources of social support are just as important to your recovery as medical and surgical interventions.

There is also communal dimension to emotional healing. No one experiences heart disease alone. True, you are the one who has high blood pressure or has survived a heart attack—but your whole family has been affected in some way. For that reason, we'll also include advice in this chapter about how your family can cope more effectively with heart disease.

■ The Emotional Impact of Heart Disease

Negative emotions such as anger, hostility, and depression all contribute to heart disease, as we discussed in Chapter 2, but it turns out they also come into play afterward. A heart attack—or even the discovery that you are at risk for one because you have high blood pressure, elevated cholesterol, or some other risk factor—may leave you feeling vulnerable. You may be asking: "Why me?" "Why now?" "What happens next?" In the days and weeks following a cardiac event, it is common to feel anxious, depressed, and stunned. This may be reflected in the self-portrait you created in Chapter 1. (See page 10 for a look at some of our patients' self-portraits.)

Recovery is a process, involving emotional as well as physical changes. People who are diagnosed with any serious illness, including heart disease, typically go through five stages similar to what people experience at the end of life. The first stage is denial and is characterized by shock and numbness: "Oh, no, not me!" or "This can't be happening." The next step involves anger: "Why me?" It is common during this stage to blame someone or something (your spouse or significant other, a doctor, God, past behaviors) for causing the current predicament. Then comes bargaining: "If I stop smoking or eat better, maybe this will go away." The fourth step is depression, when a person acknowledges what has happened but is sad about it. Typically during this stage, a person will feel tired, highly emotional, sometimes victimized. The final phase is acceptance.

Dr. Elisabeth Kübler-Ross, a Swiss psychiatrist, first identified these five stages of grief experienced in her seminal book, *On Death and Dying.* In the years since its publication in 1969, other theorists have applied her model to the process people go through when dealing with other significant traumas, such as death of a loved one, loss of a job, and diagnosis of a serious illness.

All this can make for an emotional maelstrom, especially since people go through various stages of the process at different times and the stages sometimes come in modified order. So you may feel depressed about your heart attack before you feel angry, or you may find yourself bouncing back and forth between the various stages. That's normal, but it can be unsettling. To further complicate matters, your loved ones may be at a different stage in the emotional process than you are. Your spouse may be at the bargaining stage, for instance, while you are depressed. "If only you'd quit that job sooner, this wouldn't have happened," your spouse might say to you. "I don't want to deal with this right now," may be your reply. To handle such situations it may be more helpful to understand the grieving process as a circle rather than a linear progression.

Whatever stage you are at, it is likely that your once-cohesive view of yourself and the world has fallen apart. Whereas once you felt healthy, now you feel ill. Whereas once life was predictable, now it has become unpredictable. In this situation, healing requires more than just taking medications; it requires regaining a sense of your self and what you value in life.

As you think about recovery, then, you not only have to consider getting better physically, you also have to think about getting better psychologically. To some degree, that means trying to put your vulnerable self back together again. Every step of this process involves intense emotions. First, you must acknowledge and deal with this new feeling of vulnerability. You may grieve the loss of your former carefree self and have to reevaluate your priorities and goals. As you embrace a new sense of yourself, you may

---

TABLE 10

CYCLE OF EMOTIONS ASSOCIATED WITH LOSS

Typically people go through a variety of emotions as they struggle with a significant loss, and these may not occur in linear fashion.

EVENT OCCURS
You have a heart attack.

↓

DENIAL AND SHOCK
Why me? This can't be happening.

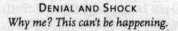

ACCEPTANCE
I've got to take each day at a time.
Lots of people survive heart attacks.
I'll change what I can about my behavior.

ANGER AND BLAME
Why didn't my doctor see this coming?
I shouldn't have eaten so much red meat.
I knew I was under too much stress at work.

DEPRESSION
I'm too young to be sick.
My life is over.
There's nothing I can do.

BARGAINING
I'll never eat red meat again.
I promise to exercise every day.
I'll go for regular checkups.

---

also find that you redefine your relationships with other people. The final step toward healing begins when you undergo a process of transformation, weaving the various strands of your life (physical, psychological, social, spiritual, and behavioral) into a new cloth.

It is normal to feel anxious, fearful, and depressed while going through this process. Eliciting the relaxation response, as we described in Chapter 3, is a good way to calm yourself and restore a sense of mental balance. As you continue to work toward recovery, though, you will also find it useful to reach out to other people. That is why finding sources of social support is so important to the healing process.

SIDEBAR 21

JOHN WAYNE NO MORE

On June 17 at 9 A.M., my neck cramped me bad.
I ignored it, as men are prone to do.
Then my stomach, too, felt bad.
I thought: I'll ice the neck to feel cool.

Thought the pain was due to food.
Poorly chosen through the day.
But nay, my friends, 'twas not to be.
Demons were headed my way.

Take Tums, I thought, and soon you'll be fine.
You're John Wayne, we all knew.
Nay, nay, my friends, 'twas not to be.
Demons were headed my way.

Round midnight same day, pain is in control.
Thought for sure I'd chased those demons away.
Like barnacles they clung, refusing to leave.
The demons were here to stay.

Blood pressure taken to see where I stood.
My bride insisted so we'd know.
Shocked to find the readings had fallen.
We thought, uncomfortably low.

Call the hospital, she wisely urged.
Let's see what the pros will say.
Much as she thought, they urged me to come in.
But never did I think I would stay.

EKG me they did! I scoffed at the test.
This John Wayne's never had a problem in his chest.
Very shortly they told me I'd had an MI.
Couldn't believe it! ME? An MI?

You're not going to keep me tonight, are you, doc?
You betcha we are, so stop watching the clock.
Three hours later there's a tube in my heart.
Three hours later, four stents in my heart.

John Wayne I'm not, just a regular guy.
Come to think of it, even Big Duke had an MI.
Lying in the hospital, invincible no more.
Wondering what now my life had in store.

—*a former patient in the MBMI Cardiac Wellness Program*

■ Finding People to Count On

Where do you normally find your primary source of social support? Many people answer "spouse," "friends," or "family." Certainly these are key components of social support, but there are others—and these less obvious sources could prove invaluable following a cardiac event.

Although we socialize with many people and in different arenas, true social support goes well beyond casual encounters and conversations. Social support is a bit like a shelter, built of many different planks of wood. It consists of emotional, physical, psychological, social, and spiritual buffers that provide comfort as you encounter the stresses of life. This "shelter" can grow stronger or weaken, depending on a number of variables. The strength of your social support depends on the number of people who provide you with emotional support, the quality and function of that support, and the frequency with which you utilize that support.

The exact mix of what constitutes social support is different for everyone. Your network of social support may consist of family, friends, and coworkers. It may also include people who belong to clubs you've joined (gardening, quilting), fellow sports team members, and people who attend your place of worship. Human beings are multifaceted. It is likely that your support comes from many sources.

To identify your particular sources of social support, ask yourself the following questions:

1. What types of supports do I have?
2. Do I count on different people for different types of support?
3. How has support been helpful or not helpful to me?
4. Whom can I count on to provide me with emotional support?
5. How does it make me feel to talk about my feelings?
6. How often do I take time to connect emotionally with another person?

Once you are diagnosed with heart disease, the nature of your "shelter" may change. People who were once your primary sources of support, such as your spouse or significant other, may not be able to provide the comfort you need (especially if they are dealing with their own emotions about your situation). You may find that your loved ones become overly protective, constantly asking you how you feel or suggesting that you should take it easy. Or you may find the opposite: that they withdraw and become distant.

Any serious illness tends to change your relationships with

others and overall family dynamics. Among possible changes, it can exacerbate underlying issues in your relationships that have not been resolved. Think about people you know and ask yourself these questions:

1. How has my heart disease changed my relationship(s)? Are they stronger? Weaker?
2. What has it been like for my family?
3. Has my family been able to make changes with me?
4. Has that helped or not helped?

As you think about your answers to these questions, it may become clear that some people are able to provide emotional support, while others cannot. To find necessary support, you may need to reach out to new people, such as members of a support group, who will help you during the healing process.

To broaden your network, see if you can name a source of support for each of the following categories. If you can't, try to come up with *potential* sources.

Emotional   (examples: significant other, friends, children)
Physical   (examples: family members, physician)
Psychological   (examples: best friend, therapist)
Social   (examples: gardening club, golf buddies)
Spiritual   (examples: church, synagogue, mosque, nature, spiritual readings)

The goal in building new networks of social support is to identify people with whom you have something in common. Your interactions with them can go beyond the small talk that dominates much of our days. Think about where you can meet people who have similar interests and values to yours and with whom you will feel comfortable opening up.

You might try this homework assignment we give to participants in our Cardiac Wellness Program:

1. Think about how you can develop social support if you do not have any right now.
2. Set yourself the goal to reach out to someone over the next week.

Of course, reaching out to people in an emotionally meaningful way—whether they are new acquaintances or old friends—requires that you open up emotionally. That can be difficult at first and involves self-disclosure, an honest look at the walls you may have built up to protect yourself.

SIDEBAR 22

SPOUSAL SUPPORT CAN HELP

Learning that a loved one has heart disease is very difficult for everyone in the family. A spouse or significant other, however, often bears the brunt of providing emotional support. The following five tips will help you reduce your stress level so that you can support your loved one when he or she needs it.

- *Take care of yourself:* Remember to eat healthy meals and exercise regularly so that you can maintain your own health and energy.
- *Acknowledge your emotions:* It's perfectly normal to feel scared, angry, and resentful at times (more on this later in the chapter).
- *Empower yourself:* Read about heart disease; seek out support groups for family members.
- *Focus on the person:* Your loved one is a person, not a disease. Take time to talk about issues other than heart disease.
- *Hugs help:* Physical intimacy and sex are valued components of most relationships. Most people can resume normal relationships after a heart attack. Ask your health care provider if you have specific concerns.

■ Self-Disclosure: Opening Up

It is a sad fact of modern life that we often spend more time thinking about external barriers than internal ones. We fret in stalled traffic, worried that the wall of cars ahead of us will prevent us from reaching an appointment on time. We dream of relaxing vacations but wonder if lack of money will prevent us from taking one. Yet sometimes the most significant barriers in life are not external (traffic, lack of money) but internal (low self-esteem, emotional walls).

Try to identify your own internal barriers by doing the following exercise on self-disclosure, which we also use in our Cardiac Wellness Program. In our classes, we advise that patients sit down with someone they don't know well, but if you feel more comfortable you can do this with a friend or even by yourself. The point is to think about the questions and then answer them as honestly as possible.

Write the following four questions down on separate slips of paper, and place them in a bag. Then pick one of the slips out of the bag, and answer the question written on it.

1. In what ways am I good to myself? How am I not good to myself?
2. During my life, in what ways has my heart been broken?
3. How have I gained from a loss in my life?
4. Have I placed walls around my heart? What are they?

After answering the question, take a deep breath and think about the experience of answering it. Was it hard? Did you find the process cathartic at all? Now that you've answered one question, go through each of the rest.

If you are like many of our patients, you may find it difficult to do this exercise at first. It requires that you recognize and acknowledge internal barriers you have built over time to protect yourself from being hurt. Yet it is likely that these same barriers also prevent you from reaching out to people in a way that is emo-

SIDEBAR 23

TIPS FOR HEART-HEALTHY COMMUNICATION

People who care about you may be feeling the same shock and stress that you do. Your heart disease may be forcing them to confront your mortality—and their own—for the first time. Some may deal with this by pestering you constantly about your health; others may simply disappear, avoiding you (and their fears) altogether. To cope:

- Understand that this is difficult for everyone.
- Don't be afraid to establish limits, especially if you need time to recover your emotional or physical energy. You may want to limit the number and duration of visits from friends, for instance.
- Let your spouse know that, when you are together, you want to talk about more than heart disease.
- Encourage family and friends to share their concerns with you, but remind them that you are the person ultimately responsible for your own health.
- Ask your health care provider for a referral to support groups that include family and friends.
- Share books and articles about heart disease with family and friends if you think that this will help them to understand your situation better.
- Tell loved ones what you need (or don't need) in the way of support; sometimes they don't know.

tionally rewarding. The first step in overcoming such internal barriers is to simply acknowledge that they exist.

■ Journaling: A Tool for Emotional Healing

Sometimes well-intentioned friends and family will advise you not to think about your heart disease or not to worry about life's events. Research indicates, however, that expressing negative emotions is better for your health than repressing them.

One way you can do this is by journaling. Many people keep diaries, but journaling involves a different process. All too often in diaries, people record the details of everyday, inconsequential events. Journaling involves much more: confronting painful realities, hard choices, and strong emotions. Journaling helps a person burrow into the depths of the soul. It's hard work, but many people find that the effort is worth it.

Much work on the healing power of journals has been done by Dr. James Pennebaker, a psychology professor at the University of Texas in Austin. In the late 1970s, Pennebaker began researching whether people who express their innermost thoughts and fears are healthier than people who do not. Pennebaker concluded that writing about traumatic events can help people to deal with the negative emotions associated with those events. People not only felt better when they wrote, their health actually improved.

In one early study, for instance, Pennebaker asked a group of student volunteers to write about superficial, nonemotional events for fifteen minutes a day, for four days. Another group wrote about traumatic incidents for the same amount of time. To focus the research further, Pennebaker divided the trauma group into three subgroups: One wrote about only the facts of the event, another wrote about only the emotions it caused, and a third wrote about both details and emotions. The researchers then determined the overall health of the student participants by comparing the number of visits they made to the student health center in the months before and after the experiment. The students also filled out questionnaires about their mood several months after the experiment ended.

Students who wrote about traumatic events reported feeling happier after the exercise than students who wrote about trivial events. When the researchers analyzed the data further, they found that participants had to write about both facts and feelings to achieve benefit. In the months following the experiment, those who had written in detail about traumatic events and explored the emotions involved in those events made 50 percent fewer visits to the health center than other students. Those who had written only about emotions or only about factual details visited the health clinic just as frequently as those who wrote about superficial topics.

In the decade since that first study, Pennebaker has taken the research even further. Working with different colleagues, he has concluded that journaling improves health in people with other medical conditions, including arthritis and chronic pain. An analysis of blood samples from participants in some studies revealed that journaling increases levels of certain immune system cells, thereby bolstering the body's natural healing powers.

More recently, Pennebaker devised a computer software program to analyze the words that were used most frequently in the journal entries. He found that people who used words mostly conveying positive emotions (such as *happy, laugh*), along with a moderate number of negative words *(sad, angry),* experienced the greatest improvement in health outcome after journaling. This suggests, he says, that those people are acknowledging problems without dwelling on them. Even more impressive, however, was the relationship between use of cognitive words *(understand, realize, because)* and recovery. People who used few of these words when they began journaling, but used many of them by the end of three or four days, tended to have better mood, health, and life outcomes than did people who used relatively few cognitive words.

Pennebaker theorizes that the people who are most likely to benefit from journaling are those who construct stories and narratives, gradually moving from expressing raw emotion to learning something from an experience or putting it in perspective. It is almost as if the physical act of writing helps the brain to process a traumatic event and then move on.

■ How to Write

Based on Pennebaker's research and our own clinical experience, we've found that journaling offers a good way to process negative events and emotions. The first step is to regard a journal as more than just a place to record events. It can be used as a tool to take stock of your life. A journal can also help you change your thoughts and feelings about a situation. Try the following assignment, which we use in our Cardiac Wellness Program:

Sit for fifteen to twenty uninterrupted minutes and write about:

1. Any life crisis you have encountered. (It can be related to your heart disease or high blood pressure but does not have to be.)
2. Your feelings and emotions concerning this crisis.

Repeat the exercise, preferably writing about the same crisis, for three to four days in a row. As you do this exercise, keep the following in mind:

Pick an important topic: Write about a stressful event, but it doesn't have to be the most damaging thing you've confronted in your life. Think about an experience that you've been mulling over, trying to resolve. Writing may help you do so. Or think about something you would like to discuss but that embarrasses you too much.

Write continuously: Pick a time when you won't be interrupted because the goal is to write continuously for fifteen to twenty minutes, without taking your pen off the paper or your fingers off the keyboard. Don't worry about penmanship (or typos, if you are typing). In this way, you will access your innermost thoughts and prevent your "inner editor" from stopping you midstream.

Write for yourself: Although you may write your entry with a particular audience in mind, and some people even write their entries in the form of letters to other people, keep the results private. Writing for yourself is the only way to ensure that you don't start shaping the narrative to avoid judgment from someone else.

Expect to feel something: As you do this exercise, you may initially feel negative emotions surface such as depression, anxiety, or sorrow. Fortunately these emotions usually dissipate within a short time. In the long term, most of our patients feel happier and more at peace—an outcome borne out by Pennebaker's studies, which find that the beneficial effects of journaling last up to six months after people finish writing their entries.

Most of our patients have found journaling to be an effective tool in dealing with emotions. As you try the journaling exercise on your own, ask yourself the following questions:

1. Were you surprised about what you wrote?
2. Did the crisis affect your family or relationship?
3. Has any opportunity come out of this crisis for you or your family?

We recommend that, to get the most out of journaling, our patients spend time writing about the same crisis for two to three days in a row. The repetition seems to help in the self-discovery and healing process.

■ Writing Your Road Map

Illness is a journey. Many of our patients say that having a heart attack or stroke made them feel very vulnerable but that it also provided them with an opportunity to reexamine their life. One woman, who suffered heart damage as a result of treatment for cancer, said she was grateful for her illness because it made her appreciate life.

Of course, reaching that level of perspective takes time. One of the most useful exercises you can do, in terms of emotional healing, is to create a map that reflects your journey in life and where you think you would like to go next. We call this the "Writing Your Road Map" exercise. Here's how you do it:

1. Find or buy some poster board.
2. Use the left-hand side of the poster board to depict the minor and major events that have shaped your life, both in a positive and negative way. If you do not want to work in a linear left-to-right fashion, you can designate any third of the poster board for past events.
3. Use the middle of the poster board (or another third of the space) to depict things you are currently doing—personally, professionally, spiritually, etc.
4. Use the right-hand side (or final third) to describe your future goals.

Beyond following these basic instructions, you can be as creative as you want. Some people cut pictures out of magazines and newspapers to illustrate key events in their lives. Others construct three-dimensional objects. The idea is not to win an art award but to express your own personal journey through life.

You may learn something unexpected. Our patients often tell us that they are surprised to rediscover how many positive events and people have been in their lives. Often we become so focused on the negative that we can think about nothing else. Creating your own personal road map is one way to see a bigger picture. It also will help you to focus on what really has been significant in your life, what has made a difference. Has it been work? Family? Spouse? Friends? Volunteer activities? Pets? It could be any one of these—or all of them.

There is no right or wrong way to draw your road map. The idea is to focus on what matters to you, what events have shaped your life, and then use that knowledge to think about where you would like to go in the future. Happy journey!

EXAMPLES OF ROAD MAPS

The following list may provide you with some ideas about how to write your own road map. These are descriptions of road maps created by some of our patients in the Cardiac Wellness Program.

Food pyramid: You're probably familiar with the FDA food pyramid, which provides advice on what to eat. Some of our patients create life pyramids, with past events forming the bottom rows (smoking, eating fast-foods, stressful life events), current events in the middle

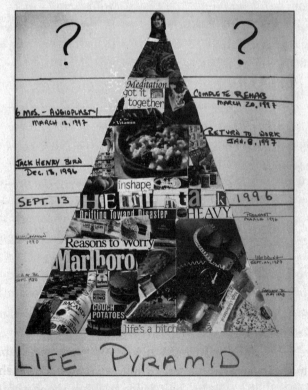

Figure 20: Sample road map

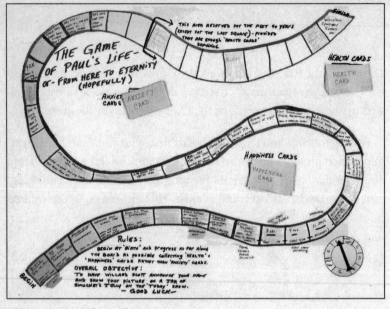

Figure 21: Sample road map

(heart attack, getting into shape, eating well), and future goals on top (appreciating the small things, time with family, meditation).

Game board: Other patients created their road maps in the form of a board game (like Chutes and Ladders). See the sample road map we have provided. Along the way, there were positive events such as graduation and marriage and children. Interspersed with these were negative events such as getting fired from a job, having a heart attack, or losing a parent.

Photo collage: This is a popular way to construct a road map. Patients use pictures from their album books to create the life map. Most patients realize they have too many pictures for the poster board and have to pare them down by identifying those most meaningful to them. What they often discover is that work that has taken up so much of their time has little value. It is their family and friends that matter most.

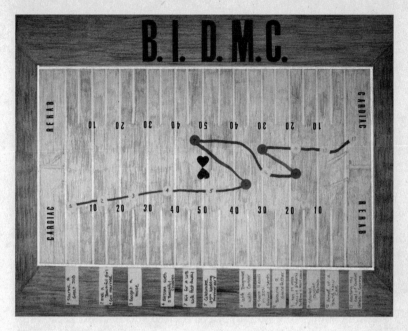

Figure 22: Sample road map

After completing her road map, one patient who had struggled for years with being overweight found out why. Food had become her best friend. It offered solace during difficult times and for her was always the focal point of family gatherings and social events. She now saw that to lose weight and keep it off, she needed to develop other interests (gardening, travel, exercise) to replace her dependence on food.

EKG: Some patients draw an EKG to depict their life map. An upward slope represents positive events, a downward slope negative events. Patients are often surprised to learn that despite the difficult times, they have experienced many positive events in their lives as well.

Name the streets: One man took the assignment literally and drew a map full of roads representing his journey. And he got creative at naming them. The roads he started out on had names like *Good Boy* and *Rat Race* because he felt that he had toed the line all his life and done what was expected. After suffering chest pain and undergoing angioplasty, his outlook changed, as did the streets he traveled. Now the roads had names like *Peace* and *Relax*.

Balance sheet: A former businessman decided to divide his life into categories, such as physical well-being, self-esteem, and finance. He then rated each, using monetary values, and added them up by decade to find out whether the decade was a net gain or loss.

Jukebox: A professional musician drew a jukebox on his poster board and added the names of songs that represented particular eras of his life. He included Yiddish folk songs he remembered from childhood, then added folk songs from the 1960s when he was a young man, and finished with his all-time favorites as he thought about his future. He also played his guitar and sang parts of the songs to convey why they represented key aspects of his life.

Color coding: One woman placed colored stickers next to each significant event she had recorded along a time line, running from left to right. The "good" events were assigned blue and purple stickers, while "bad" events were assigned orange and red. In this way, she could step back and see whether her life had been filled with mostly good things or bad.

We find that the road map exercise is often a turning point for patients. They realize they are not alone. Many patients talk of having endured past losses or difficult times and feel vulnerable when diagnosed with heart disease. However, their maps help bring to light the many contributions and successes they have achieved. Patients often say that this exercise helps them move beyond the past and look forward to a bright and enjoyable future with their families.

Chapter 6

Balance Your Plate, Help Your Heart

Dᴵᴱᴛ ʙᴏᴏᴋꜱ are perennial best-sellers in this country, yet Americans are fatter than ever before and diseases associated with obesity—including heart disease—remain the nation's leading causes of death. According to the latest statistics, three out of every five American adults are either overweight—with a body mass index (BMI) equal to or greater than 25—or obese—with a BMI of 30 or higher. (For more on BMI, see page 34.) The number of obese Americans has almost doubled since 1980, even though manufacturers have introduced a plethora of fat-free and sugar-free foods in the years since then. What is going on?

The issue is important not only because obesity is a major risk factor for heart disease, as we discussed in Chapter 2, but because whatever food you put into your mouth affects your heart. Your diet affects your blood pressure, cholesterol levels, blood clotting, and blood sugar levels. Fortunately you can prevent heart disease—or stop, slow, or even reverse its progression—by making comprehensive lifestyle changes, including following a healthy diet. In many cases, dietary changes should be tried even before medication.

Many so-called health books offer quick-fix solutions and focus on adding or subtracting particular foods from your daily diet, which can be misleading. It is not enough to give up red meat, avoid eggs, and have an alcoholic drink every day. When it comes to your heart (as well as your overall health), your whole diet matters, not just individual foods.

For instance, recent research has challenged the traditional wisdom about how to improve your overall cholesterol levels, or "lipid profile." It turns out that eggs and other foods high in dietary cholesterol do not raise cholesterol levels in your blood as significantly as red meat, restaurant fried foods, and whole milk dairy products—which are loaded with saturated and trans fats. To improve your overall cholesterol profile, you must do more than reduce total fat and avoid cholesterol-heavy foods. The National Cholesterol Education Program recommends a three-step method to reduce blood cholesterol. First, reduce intake of saturated fats, trans fats, and dietary cholesterol. Second, increase physical activity. Third, maintain a healthy weight.

Diet also affects blood pressure. The landmark DASH (Dietary Approaches to Stop Hypertension) study showed that it was possible to reduce blood pressure, even without lowering sodium intake or using medications, by consuming the right combination of foods every day. The DASH study compared three diets. One was similar to the typical American diet, with nearly 40 percent of calories coming from fat, along with one dairy product and only three servings of fruits and vegetables a day. The second more than doubled the servings of fruits and vegetables a day but otherwise resembled the typical American diet. The third DASH diet included eight to ten servings of fruits and vegetables a day, while reducing fat consumption to 27 percent of total calories and emphasizing low-fat dairy products and whole grains. The results were dramatic. Not only did the DASH diet reduce blood pressure significantly (as much as medication, in some cases), but benefits were seen almost immediately—within two weeks. A follow-up study, known as DASH-Sodium, concluded that restricting sodium intake in addition to following the DASH diet reduced blood pressure even further.

A heart-healthy diet requires making a lifetime commitment to a new way of eating and thinking about food. That may seem daunting, but in this chapter we hope to convince you otherwise. We'll provide some easy steps you can take, starting today, to begin eating in a way that is better for your heart. In the process, we'll try to cut through all the conflicting advice reported in the media and provide easy-to-follow guidelines.

■ The Basics of a Balanced Plate

If you do one simple thing every day, you will be well on the way to having a heart-healthy diet: Balance your plate.

Most Americans have an unbalanced plate at mealtime. In some cases, a huge piece of meat, poultry, or fish occupies a large part of the plate, with generous helpings of white bread, potatoes, or white rice on the side. At other times, the entire plate is filled with white pasta, which is high in calories and carbohydrates but not filling (for reasons we'll discuss later in this chapter) and completely lacking in nutrients. Vegetables and fruits, if they are on the plate at all, are added as an afterthought.

Visually, the typical American plate looks something like the top illustration on page 152. What results is an unbalanced meal that is high in calories and saturated fat, low in essential nutrients that fight chronic disease, and dominated by the types of carbohydrates that are digested so quickly that you'll soon find yourself hungry again. By eating this type of meal, you not only increase your risk for heart disease (or worsen it) but also increase your risk for other chronic diseases such as cancer.

To balance your plate, load up on nutrients and reduce the artery-clogging substances that fill a typical American plate. Start

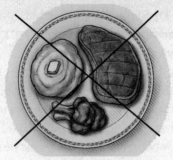

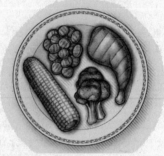

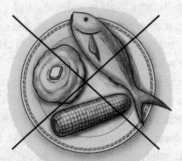

Figure 23: **Balance Your Plate**
The meat-and-starch-heavy American plate (top) and the starch-filled plate (bottom) should be avoided. Balance your plate by filling it one-half with vegetables, one-fourth with healthy protein, and one-fourth with healthy carbohydrates (middle).

by filling half of your plate with vegetables. Then fill one-fourth with a source of protein and the remaining fourth with whole grains or some other type of healthy starch. (See the middle illustration on page 152.) The beauty of this approach is that it is easy to implement, even for busy people. You don't have to measure or weigh food. Simply look at your plate to guide your food choices. Many of our patients find that having a balanced plate is one of the most effective tools for lowering cholesterol and blood pressure, and even losing weight.

One note of caution: While balancing your plate, treat certain vegetables as if they were starches. While most vegetables have about 25 calories and 5 grams of carbohydrates per serving, five vegetables—corn, peas, potatoes, plantains, sweet potatoes, and winter squash—have about 80 calories and triple the amount of carbohydrates per serving. Beans require some thought as well. Green beans are the only type of beans low in both calories and starch. All others (baked beans, black beans, pinto beans, lentils, pigeon beans, black-eyed peas, etc.) are roughly half starch and half protein. To a lesser degree than the foods on the bottom plate in the illustration, these beans are loaded with stealth starches and should be consumed in moderation.

The good news is that beans and starchy vegetables are still wonderful choices because they are loaded with nutrients that fight heart disease and other chronic conditions. We recommend that our patients substitute starchy vegetables for white rice, white bread, and other refined starches. If you enjoy corn-on-the-cob, for instance, substitute it for rice or pasta when making up a balanced plate. Beans provide additional flexibility because you can treat them as starch or protein when building a balanced plate. If you eat beans with a protein source such as chicken, treat the beans as starch (so that if you mix them with rice, the mixture should still take up only one-fourth of your plate). If you are having a vegetarian meal of beans and rice, treat the beans as protein (so that half your plate would be beans and rice, while the other

---

SIDEBAR 25

A BALANCED PLATE IS HEART-HEALTHY

With a balanced plate, you achieve five heart-healthy goals.

1. Reduce total calories because vegetables average only about 25 calories per serving (about one-third of the calories of high-protein foods and starches), which can help with body-fat loss.
2. Increase your intake of vital nutrients, such as antioxidants, B vitamins, phytochemicals, and fiber, all of which are important for heart health and cancer prevention.
3. Reduce your intake of saturated fat in order to improve your cholesterol levels and help prevent heart disease.
4. Reduce your consumption of carbohydrates to help weight loss and help prevent insulin resistance and diabetes.
5. Feel full and satisfied from a full plate of food.

---

half would be filled with low-calorie vegetables such as tomatoes, summer squash, and salad).

If you find it too difficult to create a plate that is half full of vegetables, compromise by dividing your plate into thirds, so that vegetables, protein, and starch are present in equal portions. You can even try this at breakfast. This type of plate is still better than the typical American plate. Whatever you do, try to work more vegetables into your meals: You'll be well on your way to eating in a heart-healthy way.

■ Why the Balance Tips in Favor of Vegetables

Why all this emphasis on eating more vegetables? Only about one American in four eats the recommended five servings of fruits and vegetables a day—and we consider these federal requirements a bare minimum. Not only are most vegetables low in calo-

TABLE 11

EXAMPLES OF A BALANCED PLATE

Once you get used to balancing your plate, it will become second nature. In the meantime, we've provided a few examples of how to get started.

BREAKFAST

Vegetables/Fruit	Protein	Starch
¼ cantaloupe	Skim milk	Whole-grain cereal
Mushrooms, peppers	1 whole egg (omelet)	Whole wheat toast
Fresh blueberries	Low-fat yogurt	Corn muffin with unsaturated oils

LUNCH

Vegetables	Protein	Starch
Mixed green salad	Tuna fish	Whole-grain roll
Tomatoes, onions	Black beans	Brown rice
Summer squash and tomato on side	Turkey slices	Whole-grain bread

DINNER

Vegetables	Protein	Starch
Onions, peppers, mushrooms	Chicken breast	Sweet potato
Broccoli, carrots, celery, red and green peppers	Tempeh (soy) (stir fry)	Brown rice
Mixed green salad	Salmon	Whole-grain roll

ries, but they also contain substantial amounts of fiber, which helps to slow the digestive process and modulate blood sugar metabolism, thereby helping to curb your appetite. Vegetables are also truly a "smart" food: They are chock full of nutrients and antioxidants that power the body's inborn self-repair mechanisms that help fight heart disease. (The same is true of fruits, but because these are higher in calories and sugar content, we recommend that you eat them in moderation. See Sidebar 29, page 170.)

Antioxidants include vitamins (especially vitamins C and E), minerals such as selenium, and provitamins (substances such as beta-carotene that the body turns into vitamins) that improve overall immunity and help prevent heart disease, cancer, and cataracts. Antioxidants do all this by counteracting the harmful effects of free radicals, highly reactive molecules that are first produced as by-products of normal cellular activity that involves oxygen. Free radicals are also present in the air we breathe every day, the food we eat, and the water we drink—even sunlight exposure can cause them to multiply in us. Free radicals are also abundant in cigarette smoke (another reason to quit and avoid inhaling secondhand smoke). Free radicals contribute to heart disease by turning inactive LDL cholesterol into oxidized LDL, a highly reactive substance that more easily penetrates and damages the artery wall, contributing to atherosclerosis. (For more on this process, see Chapter 2.) They may also be implicated in the development of cancer, arthritis, cataracts, memory loss, and aging.

Antioxidants serve as a wonderful defense mechanism to neutralize free radicals. Think of antioxidants as miniature armies that fight to protect your healthy cells from free radicals. The best way to build up your own protective army is to consume plenty of fruits and vegetables, which contain plentiful antioxidants. Several large epidemiological studies, conducted with both men and women, have found that people whose diets include foods that supply a lot of antioxidants are less likely to suffer from heart disease than those whose diets have insufficient antioxidant levels.

Don't try the quick fix by taking antioxidant supplements, though. For starters, supplements tend to contain one or two antioxidants, while vegetables and fruits contain dozens that act in concert to improve health. The research on antioxidant supplements has also produced mixed and sometimes worrisome results. Several studies have concluded that antioxidant supplements do not prevent heart attacks, and epidemiological research indicates that beta-carotene and vitamin E supplements may actually increase the risk of dying from one. Certain antioxidant supplements may be especially harmful if you smoke or take certain heart medications. Two large-scale studies found that smokers who took beta-carotene supplements unwittingly increased their risk for lung cancer. Antioxidant supplements also appear to undermine the beneficial effects of statins and niacin on HDL blood cholesterol levels.

Although research in this area continues, the bottom line is that you are better off eating a variety of fruits and vegetables to obtain antioxidants in their natural forms and combinations with other nutrients (all of which interact in ways we are still trying to understand). We'll go into more depth when we explain how to "color your plate" on page 169.

■ Balancing Your Plate Makes It Easy to Eat Healthy

By balancing your plate, you will turn the traditional Food Guide Pyramid on its head. That may be one of the best things you could do for the health of your heart.

The Food Guide Pyramid, developed in 1992 by the U.S. Department of Agriculture, was intended to provide people with guidance about what they should eat every day. It replaced an older precedent known as the *four major food groups*. Although the Food Guide Pyramid is more comprehensive than the earlier guide was, it has been controversial from the start, mainly because it does not distinguish between healthy and unhealthy fats or between whole-grain and refined carbohydrates. As a result, a number of alternative food pyramids exist. (For more information on the drawbacks of the FDA food pyramid, and a healthier alternative, see *Eat, Drink, and Be Healthy*, by Walter Willett, at the Harvard School of Public Health.)

Balancing your plate enables you to easily adopt healthy dietary habits without consulting a food pyramid before you sit down to eat. By filling half your plate with low-calorie vegetables, you give them the "starring" role in your diet. Other food sources become key supporting players. From a dietary point of view, both protein and fat take longer than vegetables and other carbohydrates to digest, so that you will feel full longer than if you just eat vegetables. From a biological point of view, the challenge is to choose the right types of protein, carbohydrates, and fats. To understand why some choices are healthier than others, you must first confront two of the most common—and most heart-harmful—myths about food: first, that all fats are bad; second, that all carbohydrates are good.

Myth 1: All fat is bad.
Fact: Some fats are healthy.
All fats are high in calories and have been demonized for that reason. But when it comes to heart health, not all fats are created equal—and some are even helpful when consumed in moderation. That may surprise you. It certainly contradicts many public health messages broadcast over the years with the best of intentions but with disastrous results. The "all fat is bad" message started as a way to convince Americans to cut back on fat consumption. (And to some degree, the message worked: Average fat consumption declined from 40 percent to 34 percent.) But like many well-intentioned messages, this one had unintended consequences.

The first hints about the complex relationship between fat consumption and heart disease emerged after World War II, when researcher Ancel Keys undertook the Seven Countries Study. Keys found that the higher the intake of unhealthy fat in a given country, the higher the rate of heart disease. Total fat consumption, however, did not seem to matter. The Nurses' Health Study provides further evidence that substituting healthy fats for unhealthy ones should significantly reduce your risk of dying from heart disease. Consuming certain fats may be even better for you than eating too much food high in carbohydrates. Substituting 80 calories' worth of healthy fats for 80 calories of carbohydrates daily will reduce your risk for heart disease by 30 to 40 percent.

Other evidence for the beneficial effects of fat comes from a study of the "Mediterranean diet," which consists of whole grains, plenty of vegetables and fruits, an emphasis on fish and poultry rather than red meat, and liberal use of olive oil. Among other attributes, the diet is low in unhealthy fats and rich in healthy ones. In one study, researchers found that following this diet reduces deaths from an array of causes by a stunning 70 percent.

Suffice it to say that decades of research now show that fats can be friends as well as foes. We'll explain why below, but for practical advice on how to consume proportionately more heart-friendly fats while reducing consumption of "bad" fats, see Tables 12, pages 161–163; and 13, page 164.

Heart-friendly fats: The unsaturated fats—monounsaturated and polyunsaturated—are both healthy for your heart. Unsaturated fats lower both total and harmful LDL cholesterol. In the 1990s, many experts touted monounsaturated fats as the best choice because they maintained levels of helpful HDL, but the emerging consensus is that polyunsaturated fats also do this. In addition, polyunsaturated fats appear to lower total cholesterol more than monounsaturated fats. Omega-6 polyunsaturated fats, found in vegetable oils such as corn and soybean oil, are easy to find in the American diet. Consuming enough omega-3 polyunsaturated fats might be more of a challenge, but well worth the effort. Studies show that omega-3 fats reduce your risk for heart attack and sudden cardiac death. Although the protective mechanisms are not fully known, it appears that omega-3 fats help the heart by decreasing the risk of blood clotting, maintaining a steady heartbeat, and improving cholesterol levels. A large Italian study concluded that lifesaving benefits may take effect as quickly as three to four months after regular consumption of omega-3 fats begins. Although the omega-3 fats are often referred to as *fish oils* because they are prevalent in fatty fish, that is something of a misnomer because some nuts, seeds, and oils also contain them. (See Table 13, page 164, for advice on how to get enough omega-3 fats.)

Fats that are heart foes: Both saturated fats and trans fats are heart-toxic; they increase your LDL cholesterol level and clog your arteries. While it may be impossible to avoid these fats completely, you should try to reduce consumption as much as possible. Theoretically, we don't even need to consume saturated fat because our body can make its own supplies, either by converting unsaturated fats into saturated fats or by drawing on the fat stored in muscle and fatty tissue. Whenever you are able, choose foods with any of the healthier fats we've just described rather than foods laden with saturated or trans fats.

The saturated fats contained in butter and whole milk dairy products are the worst in terms of raising levels of harmful LDL cholesterol. Those in red meats and other beef products boost LDL slightly less—but still more than is healthy. (Some good news: Chocolate boosts LDL the least of all saturated fats. That means you can occasionally indulge in a piece of chocolate or two; just don't overdo it.) While most liquid oils contain a mixture of saturated, monounsaturated, and polyunsaturated fats, try to avoid the so-called tropical oils (including palm oil and coconut oil), which contain the highest percentage of saturated fats.

Trans or hydrogenated fats are essentially man-made saturated fats. Trans fats are made by taking a liquid unsaturated oil and bubbling hydrogen gas through it to make the fat harden at room temperature. Like saturated fats, they increase LDL, and they also lower HDL levels and increase triglycerides. Not only are these fats bad for your heart, but recent studies have concluded that they may increase your risk for cancer. The prestigious Institute of Medicine recently recommended that people consume as little trans fat as possible.

Unfortunately, trans fats are abundant in the typical American diet. Deep-fried restaurant foods, such as fried seafood platters, fried chicken, French fries, and doughnuts, are loaded with trans

TABLE 12

GOOD FATS, BAD FATS

Consume more of the heart-healthy monounsaturated and polyunsaturated fats and less saturated and trans fats. Don't go overboard, though. All oils are 100 percent fat and contain about 14 grams of fat and about 125 calories per tablespoon—so they carry quite the caloric punch. Limit consumption of oils to one to two tablespoons daily to avoid weight gain. Nuts and avocados contain healthy fats but are also high in calories. Limit consumption of nuts to one-fourth cup or less (without the shells) a day; eat no more than one-half to one avocado a day.

Type of Fat	Major Sources	Recommendations

Healthy fats: Monounsaturated and polyunsaturated	Monounsaturated fats:
	• Olive oil
	• Canola oil
	• Peanuts, peanut oil, natural peanut butter
	• Avocado
	• Hazelnut oil
	• Macadamia nuts
	• Rice bran oil
	• Almonds and natural almond butter
	• Cashews
	
	Omega-3 polyunsaturated fats:
	• Flaxseeds
	• Fatty fish:
	  • Salmon
	  • Mackerel
	  • Bluefish
	  • Lake trout
	  • Sardines
	• Yellowfin or bluefin tuna steaks (fresh)
		Vary your sources to ensure you are getting a good mixture of monounsaturated and polyunsaturated fats.
		
		Pay special attention to omega-3 and omega-6 fats, as these provide essential fatty acids your body can't make on its own. (To find more on omega-3 fats, see Table 13, p. 164.
		
		Suggestions:
		Use the oils to stir-fry food or make salad dressings.
		Eat more avocados and listed nuts.
		Eat more fish, especially fatty fish.

(continued on next page)

Type of Fat	Major Sources	Recommendations
	Omega-6 polyunsaturated fats: • Sunflower seeds or oil • Sesame oil • Corn oil • Safflower oil • Soybean oil (vegetable oil) • Walnuts • Pistachio nuts	

Unhealthy fats:
Saturated and trans fats
	Saturated fats:
	• Dairy products:
	  • Butter
	  • Ice cream
	  • Whole milk
	  • 2 percent milk
	  • Cheese
	  • Yogurt that is not labeled "nonfat" or "low-fat"
	• Animal sources:
	  • Beef
	  • Veal
	  • Lamb
	  • Pork (except tenderloin)
	  • Poultry skin
	• Plant sources:
	  • Coconut oil
	  • Palm oil
	  • Palm kernel oil
	
	Trans fats
	• Deep-fried restaurant foods
	• Margarine
	• Shortening
	• Peanut butter that does not have liquid oil on top
	• Baked goods (many brands of bread, crackers, cookies, cereal, etc.)
		Limit your intake of saturated fats (measured in grams) to one-third of total fat consumption for the day or less.
		
		In its Step II diet, the American Heart Association actually recommends that you reduce saturated fat consumption to 7 percent of total fat calories or less.
		
		To reduce consumption of saturated fats:
		• Substitute fish, poultry, and nonmeat sources of protein for red meat.
		• Look for dairy products labeled "nonfat" and "low-fat."
		• Compare food labels and choose products lower in saturated fats and higher in unsaturated fats.
		
		To reduce consumption of trans fats:
		• Cut back on deep-fried restaurant food.
		• Look for margarine labeled *trans fat free*.

Type of Fat	Major Sources	Recommendations
		• Read grocery labels carefully, looking for the phrase *partially hydrogenated*. Select a different product if hydrogenated fats are listed among the first ingredients.
		• Choose natural nut butters (with oil on top) rather than solid nut butters.

fats. Trans fats are also found in many commercially baked goods, pastries, and types of margarine. Food manufacturers like to use trans fats because they are inexpensive and extend the shelf life and crispness of foods. Restaurants like them because they have a high smoking point, which makes them great for deep-frying food.

The Food and Drug Administration will require that the amount of trans fats be listed on food labels starting in January 2006. For now, all you can do is carefully scan the ingredient list for telltale words and phrases that suggest trans fats. The most common trans fat ingredients are partially hydrogenated oils, margarine, shortening, and hydrogenated oils.

Myth 2: All complex carbohydrates are good.
Fact: Whole grains and fiber are best.
It would be almost impossible to go through a day without consuming carbohydrates. Most foods, even vegetables, contain them. Traditionally, carbohydrates have been divided into two major groups: "complex" carbohydrates such as bread and pasta, and "simple" carbohydrates such as sugar and honey. The typical American gets half of his or her calories from carbohydrates. The

---

TABLE 13

OMEGA-3 FATS

Your body cannot produce omega-3 fats, so they are classified as essential fatty acids that are needed to fuel fundamental cellular processes, maintain skin quality, and improve overall immunity. Consuming sufficient amounts of omega-3 fats can be difficult since they are found in few foods. The ones we have listed are the only significant sources. Try to eat a serving or two of the following foods every day, remembering that serving sizes are small.

Source	Serving Size
Fatty fish*	3 to 5 ounces, 1 to 3 times a week
Flaxseeds**	2 to 3 tablespoons
Walnuts	2 to 3 tablespoons
Canola oil	2 teaspoons to 1 tablespoon
Soybean oil (or vegetable oil)	2 teaspoons to 1 tablespoon

---

* See list in Table 12, page 161. Canned fish contains large amounts of sodium; if possible, choose fresh fish.

** Flaxseeds contain five times the essential fats of any other nut, seed, or oil. Grind them in a handheld coffee grinder to maximize absorption in intestines. (Refrigerate after grinding them.) Sprinkle on cereal, yogurt, salads, or in homemade shakes. Flaxseeds are very flat, brown, and tiny, found in health food stores only. If you don't grind them, you risk swallowing them whole and having them pass through your body without much digestion or absorption.

---

problem with this is that the most popular carbohydrates in this country, such as white bread, white rice, and potatoes, are digested quickly and affect your body and blood sugar levels the same way as eating sugar straight from the bowl.

To understand why this happens, think about such carbohydrates from the perspective of your digestive tract, which transforms what we eat into energy our bodies can use. When you digest food, all carbohydrates break down into sugar (glucose) that

---

BUTTER OR MARGARINE?

Margarine is no better than butter. Margarine is high in trans fat and butter is high in saturated fat—so they're about equally unhealthy. Light and low-fat butter and margarine are good choices because they have about one-third the calories and saturated or trans fat of their regular-fat alternatives. Look for products with 5 grams of total fat or less or for trans fat–free varieties. Choose light, low-fat, or trans fat–free products packaged in tubs over any type of stick margarine or butter. If you are reluctant to switch to a low-fat alternative, use butter and margarine sparingly.

---

can enter the bloodstream, but some break down more quickly than others. That's why most dietitians today talk about carbohydrates in terms of their "glycemic index," the rate at which blood sugar rises after you eat. Carbohydrates with a high glycemic index, such as white bread and potatoes, quickly put you on a blood sugar roller coaster. They create a spike in blood sugar that, in turn, triggers a surge of insulin. As insulin levels rise, your body is able to absorb the glucose circulating in your bloodstream; some of it fuels the work of cells, but much of it is stored away in fat cells. As the glucose enters the cells, your blood sugar levels plummet, making you want to eat again. Many dietitians now believe that one reason Americans have grown so fat is that they are overeating the wrong type of carbohydrates (often with the intention to reduce fat consumption) and have unwittingly become riders on the blood sugar roller coaster. Ride the blood sugar roller coaster too often, and you may develop insulin resistance, so that tissues in your body become deaf to insulin's call to absorb sugar and blood sugar levels remain abnormally high. This can lead to Syndrome X, a constellation of heart-risky disorders that includes abdominal obesity, diabetes, high blood pressure, elevated choles-terol, and elevated triglycerides. (One study estimated that Syn-drome X doubles the risk for high blood pressure and triples the risk for heart disease.) To add insult to injury, the blood sugar roller coaster seems to affect overweight people most, by causing unhealthy changes in HDL and triglyceride levels and increasing risk for heart attack.

To get off the blood sugar roller coaster, eat healthy carbohy-drates such as whole-grain products, beans, and vegetables. These foods tend to be low on the glycemic index. They are digested more slowly, so that blood sugar levels rise and ebb more slowly, exerting a similar moderating effect on insulin levels. (You will get even better results with your blood sugar if you combine whole grains with an unsaturated fat or protein.) You will feel sat-isfied longer while obtaining more nutrients and vitamins. By keeping your blood sugar levels modulated, you will also find that you are in a better mood, think more clearly, perform better at work and school, and can better maintain your energy levels throughout the day. That midafternoon fog that so many people experience after eating lunch will be a memory once you substi-tute healthy carbohydrates for those that are highly refined and combine them with a protein or healthy fat.

Slowly digested carbohydrates also tend to be high in fiber, the "rough" part of carbohydrates that is amazingly gentle on the heart. A number of studies provide evidence that consuming enough fiber every day can help to prevent heart disease and re-duce your risk of suffering a heart attack. Two large-scale studies are worth mentioning here. The Physicians' Health Study found that those who consumed the greatest amount of fiber (about 29 grams a day) were 41 percent less likely to have a heart attack than those who consumed the least (about 12 grams a day). The Nurses' Health Study documented similar results in women.

Increasing daily intake of fiber is one of the best—and easiest—ways to prevent heart disease as well as to promote other

CARBOHYDRATES AND THE GLYCEMIC INDEX

HIGH-GLYCEMIC	LOW-GLYCEMIC
Potatoes	Peas and most beans
Bananas	Fruit with skin (apples, plums, etc.)
White bread	Whole-grain breads
White rice	Brown rice
French fries	Bulgur, barley
Refined breakfast cereals	Whole-grain breakfast cereals
White spaghetti	Whole-grain pasta
Sugared soft drinks	
Sugar	

aspects of good health. (We'll show you how to have a high-fiber day on page 177.) Fiber comes in two varieties: insoluble and soluble. Insoluble fiber satiates hunger pangs and helps to regulate bowel movements, and it may reduce your risk for colon cancer. It also helps prevent diverticular disease and constipation. Soluble fiber reduces cholesterol and triglyceride levels by about 10 percent, a small but still significant effect. It may also help to regulate blood sugar, which is especially helpful for people with diabetes or Syndrome X.

■ Five Steps to a Balanced Plate

Building a balanced plate is easy. You don't have to start shopping at a health food store or buy only organic products. Just follow these five easy steps, which we will explain in greater detail in the pages that follow:

SIDEBAR 28

MAJOR SOURCES OF FIBER

SOLUBLE	INSOLUBLE
Oat bran	Wheat bran
Oatmeal	Whole wheat flour
Legumes	Whole grains (breads, cereals, etc.)
Apples	Vegetables
Barley	Fruits
Carrots	Psyllium*
Psyllium*	

---

* Found in supplements such as Metamucil and in Bran Buds cereal.

---

1. *Color your plate with vegetables:* A balanced plate begins when you fill half of it with vegetables.
2. *Pick your protein:* Choose protein sources that are low in saturated fats. Consume some unsaturated fat every day.
3. *When it comes to starch, eat rough—not refined:* Whole-grain choices are healthier than white, refined products.
4. *Drink low-calorie libations:* Liquid calories add up, so make sure you drink to your health.
5. *Be mindful of particular nutrients:* Although an overall healthy diet is your most important goal, certain nutrients are particularly heart-healthy.

With proper planning and a good eye, you can find heart-healthy foods throughout your grocery store. To get you started, we've compiled a list of foods, along with brand names, that we recommend to our patients in the Cardiac Wellness Program. (See Appendix 2: Recommended Foods.) Use our grocery list to create your own so that you can make heart-healthy selections.

STEP 1: COLOR YOUR PLATE WITH VEGETABLES

Try to eat at least three servings of vegetables a day—and double or triple that amount if possible. Fresh and frozen vegetables are the best choices, because they provide the highest concentration of nutrients. Many vegetables are now frozen in the fields immediately after being harvested, using new technology, so that nutrients are retained. Canned vegetables are less nutritious, but eating them is better than not eating vegetables at all. They are also less expensive. Rinse canned vegetables thoroughly before cooking so that you reduce the added salts, or compare food labels and buy products lowest in sodium.

Vary the colors of vegetables on your plate and you will ensure that you digest a variety of nutrients and antioxidants. The colors of fruits and vegetables are determined by the concentration of substances known as *phytochemicals,* which include antioxidants and other substances that protect plants (and the people who eat them) against disease. Phytochemicals also absorb light and contribute to pigmentation, so you can tell which antioxidants are present by looking at the color of the fruit or vegetable.

Orange vegetables, such as carrots, winter squash, and sweet potatoes, contain alpha- and beta-carotene. Red vegetables such as tomatoes contain lycopene, while red grapes and blueberries contain anthocyanins. Dark green vegetables such as broccoli and kale contain sulforaphane, isothiocyanate, and indoles. Although we are still trying to figure out how each of these phytochemicals exerts its protective effects in the body, we know consuming a variety of them helps to ensure that you will be protected against a variety of toxins. Be sure, in particular, to consume dark orange and dark green fruits and vegetables, which are loaded with antioxidants.

Vegetables also supply vitamins, minerals, and fiber. "Colorizing" your plate provides a simple way to ensure that you not only consume a variety of phytochemicals but also obtain a variety of other helpful substances.

SIDEBAR 29

WHAT ABOUT FRUIT?

Fruits and vegetables are often lumped together when it comes to dietary advice, but we recommend that you treat them separately. Fruits are loaded with nutrients, phytochemicals, antioxidants, and fiber, but they also contain natural sugars. This means they have more calories than vegetables—fruit averages 60 calories per serving—and if you eat fruit too often, or all at once, your blood sugar levels and triglycerides may rise. Eat at least two servings a day of fresh fruit, canned fruit without any syrup, dried fruit, or juice, but spread out your fruit intake throughout the day.

Increasing the number of vegetarian meals you eat every week is a great way to reduce your saturated fat and cholesterol intake. This will also add variety and flavor to your meals. Try to eat at least four balanced, vegetarian meals—two for lunch and two for dinner—each week. The key word is *balanced*. Remember to include a protein source at each meal because protein helps to fill you up. There are a surprising number of sources of vegetarian protein. In Table 14, page 175, we've included a few examples of balanced vegetarian meals to help you start thinking about how to build a balanced vegetarian plate.

STEP 2: PICK YOUR PROTEIN

Some protein sources are better than others when it comes to your heart. Red meat and dairy products made from whole milk, for instance, are high in saturated fat that harms your heart. Fatty fish and many nuts contain "good" fats that help improve your cholesterol profile. Because foods high in protein often deliver more than just protein, it's important to consider the big picture as you create a balanced plate at mealtime. We'll describe different protein options below, along with their effect (good or ill) on your heart. We recommend in general that you consider vegetarian sources of protein, such as beans and soy, which you may not have considered previously. Get creative!

Meats: You don't have to give meat up altogether if you have heart disease or are concerned about developing it, but you do have to make informed choices. Eat more fish and poultry rather than red meat, choose healthier cuts of meat, and watch portion sizes.

Red meats: Beef, lamb, veal, and pork are all considered red meat. (The one exception is pork tenderloin, which is the only "white meat" from pork and is similar to poultry in terms of fat content and calories.) Because red meat is so high in saturated fats, limit your consumption to once or twice a week. (See Sidebar 34, page 196 for portion sizes.) When choosing red meat, choose cuts with the word *round* in them (e.g., top of the round, round tips, or eye of the round). The next-leanest cuts are the loins. Buy ground beef that is at least 90 percent fat free.

When choosing hot dogs and luncheon meats, look for low-fat and vegetarian choices rather than the traditional varieties, and you will greatly reduce your intake of saturated fat and calories. Watch the sodium, though; low-fat and turkey hot dogs and sandwich meat contain about the same amount of salt as the regular choices. Vegetarian meat substitutes may be the best choices because some have only 33 to 50 percent of the sodium of regular-fat or low-fat choices.

Poultry: Chicken, turkey, and game hens are generally better choices than red meat, but only if you pay attention to what you're eating. Choose white meat, which contains less saturated fat and fewer calories than dark meat. If you substitute ground turkey for ground beef, read the food label carefully to make sure skin is not ground in with the meat, since this adds saturated fat and calories and negates any health benefits. Finally, don't assume you can eat larger portions of poultry simply because it contains fewer calories than red meat. The serving recommendations are the same for poultry (and fish) as they are for red meat. (For more on portions, see Sidebar 34, page 196.)

Seafood: When it comes to animal protein sources, seafood may be your best choice of all as long as you keep portion sizes the same as those for other meats. Fatty fish, low-fat fish, and shellfish are all good choices. Seafood is heart-healthy because it has little or even no saturated fat. The fats in some fatty fish, such as salmon and sardines, provide heart-healthy omega-3 oils (see Table 13, page 164). But even those without omega-3 fats are healthy. The Physicians' Health Study found that men who eat fish even once a week reduce their risk for sudden cardiac death by about half, as compared to men who eat fish less than once per month. The Nurses' Health Study not only found similar results in women but also concluded that the more fish consumed per week, the lower a person's risk for heart disease.

Although shrimp and squid (calamari) contain moderate amounts of cholesterol, you can eat these on a weekly basis without affecting your blood cholesterol levels significantly. They may even be better choices than red meat because they are practically free of saturated fat. Other shellfish contain less cholesterol— about the same amount as in red meats, poultry, and ordinary fish. The important thing when eating shrimp and squid is to limit portion size so that you ensure your intake of dietary cholesterol remains moderate.

Nuts: Nuts and seeds contain a lot of nutrients in small packages: They are good sources of unsaturated fats, protein, fiber, vitamins, and minerals. Just be sure to eat nuts and seeds in small quantities—about one-quarter cup or less (not including shells) a day—because they are high in calories. The best approach is to sprinkle two to three tablespoons on cereal, frozen yogurt, salads, or on stir-fries. Avoid eating nuts or seeds out of the jar, since it's so easy to overdo it. Choose natural peanut butter or other nut butters with liquid oil sitting at the top that you can mix in. After mixing the peanut butter, refrigerate it to keep it mixed. Again, watch portion sizes, since natural peanut butter has just as many calories as other peanut butters.

Eggs: There's no reason to ignore eggs when choosing a protein source, even if you are concerned about your cholesterol level. Although eggs are high in dietary cholesterol, they are low in saturated fat—and as we discussed at the beginning of this chapter, saturated fat raises blood cholesterol more than dietary cholesterol does. You can eat two to four whole eggs a week, including any eggs contained in baked products. If you are worried about dietary cholesterol, remove yolks or choose Egg Beaters, which are just egg whites with yellow food coloring and preservatives.

Beans: Beans are a great choice for protein because they are high in fiber, minerals, and vitamins. We recommend you substitute beans for meat at meals and increase the number of vegetarian meals you eat each week. To consume more beans, try beans and rice, bean soups, hummus, three-bean salad, or add beans to green salads.

SIDEBAR 30

SOURCES OF DIETARY CHOLESTEROL

Cholesterol is found only in animal products. Limit consumption to 300 milligrams a day and watch portion sizes.

Liver (3 oz)	331 mg
Egg (one whole)	215 mg
Squid (calamari) (3 oz)	200 mg
Shrimp (12 medium-size)	165 mg
Meat, poultry, and fish, excluding squid and shrimp (3 oz)	40–75 mg
Cheese (1 oz), milk, or yogurt (8 oz)	20–30 mg

Soybeans: A member of the legume family of vegetables, soybeans also provide protein—and plenty more besides. Soybeans and the soy foods made from them tend to be low in saturated fats, while relatively high in unsaturated fats, protein, fiber, and isoflavones (phytochemicals that act like a weak form of estrogen and help protect your heart). There is strong scientific evidence that soy has a beneficial effect on cholesterol levels. A meta-analysis published in the *New England Journal of Medicine* concluded that substituting soy for animal protein reduced total cholesterol, LDL cholesterol, and triglyceride levels. Although researchers have not yet determined the optimal level of soy intake, the usual recommendation is that people consume at least 25 grams of soy protein a day to help their heart. That's equal to about two-and-a-half cups of tofu. But don't fret! You can use other soy foods to reach the heart-healthy goal. The most concentrated sources of soy protein are soy protein shakes, which contain 20 to 25 grams per cup, Nutlettes Soy Cereal, which has 25 grams in a half cup, and edamame (soybean pods), which has 8 grams per cup.

Soy consumption is not only good for the heart, but it may also help reduce hot flashes, strengthen bones, and reduce the risk for some cancers. We recommend that you eat soy products in moderation; two to four times a week should be fine. Some soy products make excellent substitutions for meat at meals. If you've never eaten soy before, start with a veggie burger, but there are so many other choices. Consult our list of recommended foods for other soy food choices, which we've listed under the heading "vegetarian foods" (see pages 293 to 296 in Appendix 2: Recommended Foods).

Dairy: Low-fat or fat-free products are the best protein choices from the dairy group, since those higher in fat (made from 2 percent or whole milk) contain large amounts of saturated fats and are high in calories. We'll discuss milk along with the other beverages (see page 179), but remember that it can also be used as protein when creating a balanced bowl of cereal.

TABLE 14

BALANCE YOUR VEGETARIAN PLATE

The easiest way to balance your plate while eating vegetarian is to include a food from each of the following three categories. (Don't forget the protein.) This may take some planning at first, but soon it will become second nature. We've left several lines blank so that you can add your own ideas.

Protein Source	Vegetable or Fruit	Grain or Starch
Skim milk	Strawberries	Whole-grain cereal
Veggie burger	Steamed broccoli	Whole wheat hamburger bun
Natural peanut butter	Banana	Whole wheat bread
Black beans	Tomato	Brown rice
_____	_____	_____
_____	_____	_____

Sources of vegetarian protein:
  Dairy: skim or 1 percent milk, low-fat or nonfat cheeses and cottage cheeses, and low-fat or nonfat yogurt
  Beans: all beans except green beans
  Other sources:
    Hummus, which is made from chickpeas
    Soy products (including tofu, tempeh, soy protein shakes, veggie burgers, and soy milk)
    Eggs or egg whites
    Nuts and natural nut butters (including peanut butter and almond butter)
    Seeds

Yogurt: Like beans, yogurt is a versatile food; you can eat it as part of a regular meal, as a healthy snack (which we'll discuss in the next chapter), or even as dessert. Yogurt not only provides many nutrients, but certain brands also contain helpful bacteria that aid digestion. (Look for the phrase *live cultures* to make sure you are getting these healthy bacteria.) Choose low-fat or nonfat yogurt, and compare labels to find brands lowest in sugar and saturated fat.

Cheese: Many types of cheese are now available in low-fat versions, and while some taste like plastic or rubber, several are tasty. (See pages 285 and 286 in Appendix 2: Recommended Foods for low-fat cheeses.) Watch sodium content when selecting cheese, and choose products that have about 3 to 4 grams of fat and no more than 200 milligrams of sodium per ounce. If you are unwilling to change to low-fat cheese, consume smaller portions of the regular-fat variety.

STEP 3: WHEN IT COMES TO STARCH, EAT ROUGH—NOT REFINED

As we discussed earlier in this chapter, the best choices for starch on your balanced plate are low-glycemic, fiber-rich foods that supply carbohydrates that are digested slowly and help modulate blood sugar. Unfortunately, an astounding four in five Americans eat less than one serving a day of these "good" carbohydrates. To get smart when it comes to starch, reduce your consumption of refined foods, especially products made of white flour, and get rough: Eat more whole-grain products and vegetables.

Whole grains include brown rice, whole wheat bread, and whole-grain cereals and pasta. Make sure the word *whole* is on the list of ingredients. Many so-called healthy products list "wheat flour," which is just another name for refined white flour. Whenever possible, substitute whole-grain products for white rice, white bread, and fiber-free cereals such as cornflakes or Rice Krispies. You can also "think outside the rice box" by trying grains like kasha, bulgur, and quinoa.

Eating more whole grains will help you obtain adequate amounts of fiber. Sadly, most Americans eat only 12 grams of fiber a day, which is half the amount they need for the protective benefits documented in research studies. To consume adequate fiber, choose cereals that have at least 3 grams of fiber per serving

TABLE 15

HOW TO HAVE A HIGH-FIBER DAY

To protect your heart, consume about 25 grams of fiber a day. Just a few adjustments in your diet make it easy to achieve that goal.

Low-Fiber Day	(grams of fiber)	High-Fiber Day	(grams of fiber)
Cornflakes (1 oz)	0.3	Kashi (1 oz.) (cereal)	8.0
Skim milk (½ cup)	0.0	Skim milk (½ cup)	0.0
Orange juice (½ cup)	0.5	Banana (1 medium)	2.8
Breakfast total	**0.8**	**Breakfast total**	**10.8**
Turkey (2 oz)	0.0	Turkey (2 oz)	0.0
White bread (2 slices)	0.8	Whole wheat bread (2 slices)	2.8
Peach (1 medium)	1.7	Apple (1 medium)	3.7
Skim milk (1 cup)	0.0	Skim milk (1 cup)	0.0
Lunch total	**2.5**	**Lunch total**	**6.5**
Chicken breast (4 oz)	0.0	Chicken breast (4 oz)	0.0
Summer squash (1.5 cup)	4.2	Broccoli (1.5 cup)	6.9
White rice (²/₃ cup cooked)	1.0	Brown rice (²/₃ cup cooked)	3.0
Dinner roll (1)	0.9	Carrots (½ cup)	2.3
Skim milk (1 cup)	0.0	Skim milk (1 cup)	0.0
Dinner total	**6.1**	**Dinner total**	**12.2**
Total day's fiber	**9.4**	**Total day's fiber**	**29.5**

The calorie totals for the two days are about the same, but the fiber triples to heart-protective levels on the high-fiber day.

and try to eat other fiber-containing foods throughout the day. If all else fails, try a fiber supplement, especially one that contains psyllium. If you plan to increase your fiber intake, start slowly and build over several weeks so that your gastrointestinal tract will have time to adjust, and make sure that you drink more fluids—otherwise, you may experience gastric distress or become consti-pated. Fiber absorbs fluid and softens as it moves through the digestive tract, so you'll need to drink enough liquids to make up the difference.

STEP 4: DRINK LOW-CALORIE LIBATIONS

People need fluids as well as solid food to keep healthy, and what you drink affects the health of your heart for better or worse. Yet many people forget about beverages when thinking about calorie consumption, saturated fat, cholesterol levels, and nutrients.

How much do you need to drink every day? The standard ad-vice is to consume 64 ounces of liquid a day (eight 8-ounce glasses), which is based on the need for fluids of the average per-son, who has a 2,000-calorie daily diet. Your particular need for fluids may be different, depending on your calorie needs, activity level, diet, and even where you live. If you are physically active (and if not, we hope to make you so in Chapter 8), drink more flu-ids each day. Anything besides alcohol and caffeinated beverages (which lead to dehydration) count toward the total, so you have a variety of options.

Your best choice is water. It provides your body with liquid and has no calories or additives. (Sugary drinks don't fill you up and—except for fruit juices have no nutritional value.) One recent study found that people who drink a lot of water (five or more glasses a day) were about half as likely to die from heart disease as those who drank only two glasses a day or less. (Men reduced their risk by 54 percent, women by 41 percent.) Tap water is fine (and cheap), since public water supplies in the United States are gener-ally safe and constantly monitored. If you prefer, bottled water is also fine—and some bottled-water products are flavored without additional calories. (But read the labels: Some bottled "waters" contain large amounts of added juice or sugar.)

Watch the calorie count and total carbohydrate content in sugary beverages. Restrict your intake to a 6-ounce glass of real fruit juice a day (as opposed to a flavored imitation with added sugar). If you are on heart medication, be wary of grapefruits and grapefruit juice, which changes the way some people absorb and metabolize certain drugs. (Check with your physician for details.) When it comes to milk, the best choices are skim or 1 percent, which contain fewer calories and less saturated fat than whole and 2 percent milk. This not only helps you watch your weight but also helps keep your cholesterol levels from rising. If you are lactose intolerant, try Lactaid milk, Lactaid droplets, or soy products fortified with calcium.

Consume soda and sports drinks only on occasion. Typical 12-ounce cans of sugared soft drinks such as cola, ginger ale, and root beer contain the equivalent of as much as ten teaspoons of sugar. If you insist on drinking soda, do so in moderation or choose sugar-free varieties. Many sports drinks are also loaded with sugar. The best-tasting low-calorie choices are $Fruit_2O$ and Gatorade Propel, made with sucralose (Splenda), one of the newer sugar substitutes on the market.

Need caffeine? The scientific consensus is that coffee is fine if you drink no more than one to two 8-ounce cups per day. To avoid a small spike in your cholesterol, drink coffee from a drip pot rather than an espresso maker, French press, or any other devices in which the water does not drip through a paper filter. Both green and black teas contain polyphenols, chemicals that have antioxidant properties and protect cells. If you are sensitive to caffeine, choose herbal teas and decaffeinated varieties of teas and coffees.

A number of studies have concluded that regular but moderate consumption of alcohol can protect against heart disease, probably because it raises HDL cholesterol and reduces risk for blood clots. (Moderate alcohol intake equals one drink a day for women and two drinks a day for men, where one drink is defined as a 12-ounce beer, a 5-ounce glass of wine, or a 1½-ounce shot of hard liquor.) Although red wine was initially dubbed most heart-healthy, it now appears that any type of alcohol provides the same benefits. Drink too much, however, and you'll lose most of the benefits alcohol confers. Alcohol raises blood pressure and triglyceride levels in some people, and when consumed in excess quantities can damage the heart muscle over time. It is also toxic to the liver.

STEP 5: BE MINDFUL OF PARTICULAR NUTRIENTS

As you balance your plate, try also to ensure that you get adequate amounts of nutrients for maintaining overall health. Several vitamins and nutrients are particularly good for your heart, but a few have not lived up to benefits touted on the basis of preliminary studies. Here's a brief low-down on vitamins and nutrients to pay attention to, and why.

B vitamins: All eight B vitamins are incredible workhorses. They help a number of enzymes convert food into energy, and then help transport oxygen and nutrients around the body. Three B vitamins in particular—B_6, B_{12}, and folic acid—appear to protect against heart disease, probably because they reduce levels of homocysteine, a by-product that results from your body digesting and metabolizing protein. High levels of homocysteine damage artery walls and may increase the risk for heart disease. (In the Physicians' Health Study, for instance, high levels of homocysteine tripled the chances of having a heart attack. The Nurses' Health Study found that women who consumed more than the recommended daily amount of B vitamins—either through diet alone or by taking a daily multivitamin—had the lowest risk for heart disease.) There have been conflicting findings about whether high homocysteine levels increase the risk for restenosis (a condition whereby an artery opened with a stent during angioplasty becomes reclogged and another stent has to be inserted). Some studies also suggest that regular intake of B vitamins may

---

BEAT HEART DISEASE WITH THE B'S

You can usually obtain the recommended B vitamin levels by taking a daily multivitamin or eating fortified breakfast cereals. Here are other major sources of the heart-helpful B vitamins:

B$_6$ (Aim for 1.3–1.7 mg daily.)
Meat
Nuts
Beans

B$_{12}$ (Aim for 6 mcg daily.)
Liver
Tuna
Yogurt
Cottage cheese
Eggs

Folic Acid (Aim for 400 mcg to 1 mg daily.)
Liver (Chicken contains more than three times the amount in beef.)
Beans (especially lentils, black beans, and baked beans)
Spinach (cooked)
Orange juice
Chickpeas

---

decrease the likelihood of restenosis, although—again—the jury is still out.

Ask your doctor whether you should have your homocysteine level checked. To be on the safe side, consume at least the recommended daily amounts of B$_6$, B$_{12}$, and folic acid every day, either by eating the right foods or taking a B complex or multivitamin supplement. (See the sidebar on this page for good sources of B vitamins.)

Iron: Iron helps red blood cells deliver oxygen throughout the body, which in turn helps you feel energized and alert. Iron's effect on the heart is less clear. Many studies have found that high iron levels increase the risk for heart disease, although others have contradicted this. Even so, it's good for your overall health to keep iron levels in balance, and the best way to do this is to eat the right foods. Your body carefully monitors any iron ingested from whole grains, fruits, vegetables, or supplements, and excretes unneeded quantities in urine. Unfortunately a major source of iron in the American diet, red meat, supplies iron in a way that somehow eludes your body's internal regulatory sensors. Although further research is needed, try for now to get most of your iron from foods your body can regulate, while keeping red meat consumption at moderate levels. If you take a daily multivitamin, take one without iron. The only time you should take a multivitamin with iron is if your health care provider recommends it to treat iron-deficient anemia, and even then take a supplement containing only the recommended daily amount.

Salt: To function, the human body needs only about 500 milligrams of sodium (a major constituent of table salt) a day under normal circumstances, yet the average American consumes 4,000 to 5,800 milligrams a day. Reducing that amount by at least half—to 2,000 milligrams a day—will lower blood pressure in most people.

Start by keeping track of your intake of sodium for a day or two. If it is high, begin weaning yourself away from salt by gradually reducing consumption. Most people know enough to stop adding table salt to food, but you also have to watch out for hidden salt— for example, in canned, frozen, and other processed foods, which supply about two-thirds of the sodium Americans consume every day. Fast-foods and restaurant foods are also typically high in sodium. The easiest way to start lowering your sodium intake is to eat more fresh foods and meals cooked from scratch. Try replacing some high-sodium foods with substitutes, including healthier

TABLE 16

LOW-SODIUM ALTERNATIVES

The following table lists high-sodium foods and some low-sodium alternatives.

Limit intake of these foods . . .		Eat these instead . . .	
Canned vegetables (½ cup)	122–530 mg	Fresh or frozen vegetables (½ cup)	avg = 17 mg
Sauerkraut (½ cup)	780 mg		
Sour/dill pickle (large)	1,400 mg		
Sweet pickle (large)	572 mg		
Green olives (2 medium)	312 mg		
Greek olives (3 medium)	658 mg		
Instant oatmeal (1 packet)	280 mg	Hot cereals (1 cup)	avg = 3 mg
Cold cereals (1 oz)	>200 mg	Cold cereals (1 oz)	<200 mg
Canned baked beans (½ cup)	525 mg	Dried beans/legumes (½ cup)	3 mg
Sardines canned in oil (8)	510 mg	Fresh fish (3 oz)	avg = 75 mg
Tuna, canned (3 oz)	300 mg		
Salmon, canned (3 oz)	458 mg		
Turkey roll (3 oz)	480 mg	Fresh poultry (3 oz)	avg = 75 mg
Turkey hot dog (2 oz)	808 mg		
Turkey ham (3 oz)	840 mg		
Bacon (3 slices)	303 mg	Fresh beef or pork (3 oz)	75 mg
Sausage links (3)	500 mg		
Bologna (3 oz)	1,000 mg		
Salami (3 oz)	900 mg		
Beef/pork hot dog (2 oz)	639 mg		
Ham (3 oz)	1,023 mg		
Corned beef (3 oz)	964 mg		
Canned soups (1 cup)	700–900 mg	Low-sodium soups (1 cup)	<100 mg
Dehydrated soup (1 pkg)	900–1,300 mg		
Bouillon cube (1)	1,008 mg		
Onion soup mix (pkg)	3,493 mg		

(continued on next page)

Limit intake of these foods . . .		Eat these instead . . .	
American cheese (1 oz)	337 mg	Alpine Lace cheese (1 oz)	35 mg
Cottage cheese (½ cup)	318 mg		
Feta cheese (1 oz)	316 mg		
Italian dressing (1 tbsp)	150 mg	Oil and vinegar (1 tbsp)	0 mg
Soy sauce (1 tbsp)	1,029 mg	Low-sodium soy sauce (1 tbsp)	412 mg
Salted snack foods (1 oz)	~200 mg	Unsalted snack foods (1 oz)	~65 mg
Canned tomato products, such as tomato sauce or diced tomatoes (4 oz)	~700 mg	Low-sodium tomato products, such as tomato sauce or diced tomatoes (4 oz)	~25 mg
Salt (1 tsp)	2,300 mg	Papa Dash (1 tsp)	270 mg

flavorings for salt (any herb or spice) when cooking or eating. Read food labels carefully. If salt or sodium is listed in the first five ingredients, the product is generally high in sodium. Pick another brand or a different food.

As you lower your sodium consumption, you may find that you miss the taste of salt at first. It usually takes a month for your taste buds to adjust. If you get discouraged, remember this: We *acquire* a taste for salt, we are not born with it. (Most infants dislike the taste of salt, and people develop a taste for it simply because it's so hard to avoid in our society.) Since salt is an acquired taste, it can also be de-acquired. Most people find that once they stop eating salty foods for a while, they do not miss the salt. If anything, eating something salty after reeducating your taste buds may actually turn your stomach—much like whole milk and cream tastes thick and unpleasant to people who have switched to drinking skim and 1 percent milk.

HEALTHY SEASONINGS

Any of the following condiments will add flavor and spice to your food without also adding excessive amounts of calories:

Herbs and spices	Tabasco sauce
Horseradish	Low-sodium tomato sauce or
Low-sodium ketchup	puree
Lemon, lime, and other fruit	Vinegar
juices	Wine, sherry, brandy, vermouth,
Mustard	rum
Onion and garlic powder	Tarragon
Reduced-sodium soy sauce	Sage
Worcestershire sauce	Mint
Low-sodium bouillon and stock	Thyme
Low-sodium tamari	Parsley
	Basil

Vitamin E: A few years ago, vitamin E suddenly appeared on the radar screen as a substance that could possibly offer protection against heart disease. Early studies suggested that vitamin E might prevent the oxidation process that transforms relatively benign LDL into the more volatile form that penetrates artery walls and contributes to heart disease. Some studies showed that diets rich in natural vitamin E (found in nuts and oils) might protect against heart disease. However, it is less clear whether vitamin E supplement pills offer the same protection. For now, there is not enough evidence for us to recommend that you take vitamin E supplements. (People who smoke, or people who take niacin and statins, should never take vitamin E supplements. See pages 156 and 157.)

■ Become a Balanced Cook

Our master shopping list (in Appendix 2: Recommended Foods) will help you compile your own personal list of healthy products and ingredients to buy at the grocery store. Once you get home, it's also important to pay attention to how you prepare and cook food. Otherwise, you may be adding saturated fat, cholesterol, and sodium to your balanced plate without being aware of it.

To get as many nutrients as possible, it's best to prepare foods fresh every night. If this is just not possible, try to cook ahead of time and then freeze or refrigerate portions so that you can use them during the week. When you are hungry and heading home late at night, it is reassuring to know that you have something in your fridge that is healthy and only needs to be warmed up. This may help you cut down on the number of fast-food, restaurant, and prepackaged meals you eat during the week.

Try these heart-healthy strategies in the kitchen:

- Trim fat from meat before cooking it.
- You can keep the skin on poultry during cooking, but remove it before serving, which reduces fat content and calories by 50 percent!
- When frying foods in oil, use healthy monounsaturated and polyunsaturated oils, such as olive or canola oil, rather than butter, margarine, or other oils high in saturated fats. (When baking, substitute three-quarters the amount of oil for butter and margarine).
- The best techniques for cooking are baking, broiling, grilling, steaming, poaching, boiling, and microwaving.
- Stir-frying can be healthy. In spite of its name, this cooking technique is not so much about frying as it is about steaming food. Start cooking the ingredients in a few tablespoons of oil and then add a few tablespoons of water whenever the pan dries out. Small amounts of water will create steam in an open

pan, although you can also cover the pan to enhance the steaming effect.

- Cook vegetables for five to seven minutes or less, so that they are still firm or crunchy, and you will retain most of the nutrients. This is especially true of vegetables that contain vitamin C, which is very heat sensitive.
- Substitute healthy foods for foods laden with calories and saturated fat. (See Table 17, below.)

TABLE 17

HEALTHY SUBSTITUTIONS

The foods that appear in the left column are all high in saturated fats as well as total fat. By substituting the healthier choices we suggest, you will reduce both total and saturated fat consumption (only total fat count is listed).

Instead of:	Try:	You will save:
1 strip bacon	1 tbsp imitation bacon bits	31 cal, 3 g fat, 56 mg salt
	1 oz cooked Canadian bacon	111 cal, 12 g fat
1 tbsp butter or margarine	1 tbsp healthy oil	6 g fat
1 oz cheese	1 oz part–skim milk cheese	40 cal, 4 g fat
1 oz chocolate, unsweetened	¼ cup baking cocoa + 2 tsp margarine	38 cal, 4 g fat
½ cup light cream	½ cup evaporated skim milk	132 cal, 22 g fat
1 oz cream cheese (2 tbsp)	1 oz yogurt cheese	67 cal, 9 g fat
	1 oz light cream cheese	37 cal, 5 g fat
	1 oz Neufchâtel cheese	25 cal, 3.3 g fat
1 egg	1 nonfat egg substitute or 2 egg whites	50 cal, 6 g fat

(continued on next page)

Instead of:	Try:	You will save:
1 oz cooked ground beef, regular or 25 percent fat	1 oz cooked Perdue ground turkey	34 cal, 4 g fat
	1 oz cooked extralean ground beef	10 cal, 1.5 g fat
	1 oz cooked ground tenderloin	35 cal, 4.5 g fat
1 cup whole milk or 1 cup 2 percent fat milk	1 cup skim or 1 percent fat milk	25–60 cal, 2–7 g fat
1 oz cooked sausage	1 oz cooked turkey sausage	50 cal, 5 g fat
	1 oz cooked Morningstar Farms Breakfast Links	30 cal, 4 g fat
1 tbsp sour cream	1 tbsp nonfat yogurt	20 cal, 3 g fat
	1 tbsp light sour cream	6 cal, 1.5 g fat

▪ Balance Your Plate Away from Home

The average American eats out four times a week. Maybe you grab a sandwich on your lunch break. Or perhaps at the end of the day you feel too tired to cook and decide to go out to a restaurant. Americans currently consume more than one-third of their calories outside the home, twice as many as they did thirty years ago.

You may think of eating out as something enjoyable, and it can be—but you also may be unwittingly damaging your heart. Many restaurants are notorious for serving up unbalanced plates filled with unhealthy ingredients. Portion sizes have also increased dramatically over the years, resulting in supersized foods and drinks that can supply almost an entire day's worth of calories in one meal. The U.S. Department of Agriculture estimates that restaurant meals are 20 percent higher in total fat content and 15 percent higher in saturated fat than those prepared at home. Meals at restaurants usually contain more sodium and cholesterol and less fiber and iron than homemade meals. Fortunately, you can take steps to balance your plate even when dining out. Here are some strategies that have worked for our patients:

Be prepared:
- Go into a restaurant with the attitude that the staff will try to overfeed you. Most restaurants serve extra-large portions. In spite of what your parents may have told you when you were younger, you don't have to clean your plate!
- Plan ahead of time to take some food home or send it back to the kitchen, knowing you are satisfied but did not overeat. You can even request a doggie bag when you order your meal, and place half of the meat entrée in it immediately. This technique is especially helpful if you are worried about whether you will have the willpower to stop eating halfway through.
- Choose restaurants that can accommodate your special requests.

Start with an appetizer:
- Choose low-fat appetizers such as clear soups, shrimp cocktail, or steamed clams. These will take the edge off your appetite without piling on extra calories.
- Order soup if you're especially hungry, because foods with a high liquid content tend to fill you up. (Just be aware that restaurant soups are usually high in salt content.)
- Order a salad, which will provide you with extra servings of vegetables. Ask for a clear or vinegar and oil dressing on the side and apply sparingly to avoid adding extra hidden calories.
- Ask for only one piece of bread or one roll or ask not to be served bread at all.

Think small when selecting an entrée:
- Consider ordering an appetizer as your meal.
- Split an entrée with your dining partner.

- If ordering meat, choose lean cuts (loins or rounds). Cut the serving of meat in half when it arrives at the table, and bring the uneaten half home so that you can eat it for lunch the next day.
- Order vegetarian meals more often.
- Ask for a side dish or two of the vegetable of the day, or substitute lower-calorie vegetables for potatoes.
- Look for healthy selections on the menu. Some restaurants have added such items, usually noted with a heart icon or the words *light* or *heart-healthy*.

The deal on dessert:
- Split desserts with your dining partner.
- Consider skipping dessert altogether.

Special situations:
- At Asian restaurants, if you order a stir-fried dish, ask for an extra plate and scoop the food onto the second plate, trying to leave most of the sauce behind. We estimate that, by doing without the extra sauce, you can reduce sodium intake by about half and cut out a lot of calories.
- When traveling by plane, order low-calorie or vegetarian meals ahead of time.
- At fast-food restaurants, order salads, single hamburgers, veggie burgers, grilled chicken sandwiches, or baked potatoes.

As you learn to balance your plate, whether at home, work, or dining out with friends, you should find that you not only feel better but that you are making healthy food—and enjoyable mealtimes—more of a priority in your life. In the next chapter, we'll explore how to make positive changes in your relationship with food.

Chapter 7

Improve Your Relationship with Food

MANY AMERICANS take better care of their cars than they do of their own bodies. Regular oil changes and unleaded fuel help keep a car running longer partly because they limit internal wear and tear on the vehicle. The same principle applies to your body, which is a biological machine that also requires the right fuel to function efficiently. Yet many people never pay attention to the type of fuel they put into their bodies.

Although there are many reasons for this, much of it boils down to mindless eating. Think back to your last meal. Can you even remember what you ate? (You'd be surprised at how many people can't.) Did you savor it or did you quickly shovel the food in your mouth while doing something else?

In this chapter, we'll suggest ways for you to become more mindful of what, when, and why you are eating. In order to reach this awareness you may have to improve your relationship with food. Our goal is also to help you make food more of a priority in your life, because if you pay more attention to what you eat, you will enjoy health benefits whether you already have heart disease or are trying to prevent it.

■ Eat Regularly but Eat Well

When it comes to food, the healthiest approach is to emulate birds: Eat small meals throughout the day. Instead of following the traditional three-meals-a-day approach, try reducing plate size (and portions) at breakfast, lunch, and dinner, then add one or two healthy snacks in between regular meals or at night. As long as your plate is balanced, this approach will help keep your blood sugar levels stable and supply your body with a steady stream of energy.

Healthy snacks are particularly important. Although it may seem counterintuitive, snacking actually helps reduce cravings by maintaining your blood sugar levels between meals. The key is to snack wisely. Avoid the common trap of eating nothing but carbohydrates when you snack, because carbohydrates alone (even whole grains that are high in fiber) will not fill you up, and you may find yourself gobbling down more crackers, cereal, or chips than you intended. To make your snack more substantial and filling, combine a whole-grain carbohydrate item with a protein source or a healthy fat—two types of food that take longer to digest and satisfy you longer than carbohydrates. Just make sure to consume fewer carbohydrates whenever you add a protein or fat, to keep total calories at snack-size levels. Some suggestions: Spread natural peanut butter onto two or three whole-grain crackers, or fill half a coffee mug with whole-grain cereal and then add low-fat milk. Always choose whole-grain, high-fiber carbohydrates to avoid putting yourself on the blood sugar roller coaster. (For more on this, see Chapter 6.) If you eat a healthy snack at a designated time every day, you will lessen your chances of eating candy or junk food randomly during the day. You are also less likely to become so hungry by day's end that you eat a huge dinner.

HEALTHY SNACK SUGGESTIONS

To create a healthy snack, try one of the following combinations. Or make up your own by choosing a source of protein or healthy fat with a carbohydrate.

PROTEIN SOURCES	CARBOHYDRATES
Veggie burgers (soy)	Whole-grain bread
Veggie dogs (soy)	Whole-grain bread
Low-fat cottage cheese	Fruit, whole-grain crackers, rice cakes
Low-fat cottage cheese	Baked potato
Natural peanut butter (1 tbsp)	Whole-grain bread or crackers
1 percent or skim milk	Whole-grain cereal (<5 g sugar/serving)
Low-fat or fat-free yogurt	Fruit with grapenuts
Baked tofu	Whole-grain crackers
Bean dip or hummus	Baked tortilla chips or whole-grain crackers
Low-fat dip	Raw vegetables, whole-grain crackers
1 percent or skim milk	Popcorn (popped yourself; no butter or salt)
Canned beans	Tortilla and salsa = burrito
Clear soups with beans or chicken	Whole-grain crackers
Cheese (low-fat)	Whole-grain crackers
Mozzarella cheese (<3 g fat/oz)	Whole-grain muffin and tomato slice = pizza
Skim or 1 percent milk	Carnation Instant Breakfast
Turkey, chicken, or tuna	Whole-grain bread = sandwich
Soy nuts	Dried fruits (2 tablespoons)
Nuts (¼ cup or less)	Dried fruits (2 tbsp)
Egg whites or whole egg (2–4/week)	Whole-grain toast, muffin, or bagel
Flaked tuna	Salad
Tofu salad*	Whole-grain bread

---

* *Tofu salads are usually found only at whole-food stores.*

■ Maintain a Healthy Weight

The best way to maintain a healthy weight is to make sure you ingest only as many calories as you really need every day. Balancing your plate (see Chapter 6) is a good first step, but you may also need to take a food reality check.

Determine your daily needs: Food labels typically list "percent daily values" of various food components in two columns, one for people who consume 2,000 calories a day and the other for 2,500 calories a day. Many people assume that this is the daily calorie range they should aim for. Not necessarily. The number of calories you need every day to maintain your weight and your daily requirement for particular components such as fats and carbohydrates may be different from the average—especially if you want to lose weight or either have heart disease or are trying to prevent it.

To lose weight, subtract 250 to 500 calories daily (by eliminating a candy bar or reducing portion size at meals, for example) for a one-half to one pound weight loss per week. To gain weight, add 250 calories a day. To improve your cholesterol profile and help prevent heart disease, follow the guidelines provided in Table 18, page 195.

Beware of portion distortion: Many people are surprised to learn just how small serving sizes really are. When shopping, always check serving size on food labels first, because everything that follows—calorie count, nutritional values, salt content, etc.—is based on the serving size designated on the label. Many serving sizes designated by food manufacturers—even those that produce heart-healthy food—are small and unrealistic for most people. What you consider a serving may be double or triple the size specified on the label. Therefore, determine the number of servings you realistically expect to eat in one sitting, and multiply the calories, grams, and milligrams on the food label by that number.

TABLE 18

RECOMMENDED NUTRIENT INTAKE FOR
PREVENTING HEART DISEASE

Nutrient	Recommended Intake
Total calories	Your weight in pounds $\times$ 11.4
Total fat	25 percent to 35 percent of total calories
Saturated fat	12 to 15 grams a day or less
Other fats	Consume as little trans fats as possible; make sure most of your fat calories come from unsaturated fats.
Carbohydrates	50 to 60 percent of total calories (Choose whole-grain, high-fiber sources.)
Cholesterol	Try to keep less than 300 mg a day.
Sodium	Keep less than 2,000 mg a day.
Fiber	Consume 25 grams or more a day.
Sugar	Limit sweets (candy, cookies, etc.; not fruit) to 200 calories a day.

Then you will have a better sense of what each serving you eat contains. Concentrate on total calories, saturated fat, fiber, sodium, and total carbohydrates. Then compare the numbers you come up with to the daily recommendations we've provided in Table 18, above.

Let's say the serving size listed for cereal is three-quarters of a cup; that is less than half the amount you could fit in a typical cereal bowl. If you double or triple the recommended serving size listed on the label, you should also double or triple the total calorie, fat, sugar, and sodium count. The point to consider is that labels should be used as a guide, but you need to pay attention to details. It's also good to decide on what to eat at a particular meal based on what you have already eaten that day or what you expect to eat later on. For instance, if you choose a high-calorie, high-sodium lunch, then eat a low-calorie, lower-sodium supper than you ordinarily would for balance.

SIDEBAR 34

SAMPLE SERVING SIZES

Vegetable Group (25 calories/serving)
$^1/_2$ cup of chopped, raw, or cooked vegetables
1 cup of leafy vegetables
6 fluid ounces of vegetable juice such as V8

Fruit Group (60 calories/serving)
1 small to medium piece of fresh fruit
$^1/_2$ cup of apple, orange, or grapefruit juice
$^1/_3$ cup of cranberry juice cocktail or grape juice
$^1/_2$ cup of canned fruit
2 tablespoons of dried fruit
$^3/_4$ cup of blueberries
$1^1/_4$ cup of whole strawberries

Grain Group (80 calories/serving)
1 slice of bread
$^1/_2$ cup of cooked rice or pasta
$^1/_2$ cup of cooked cereal
1 ounce of ready-to-eat cereal
1 tortilla
2 rice cakes
$^1/_2$ English muffin

Dairy Group (calories vary)
1 cup of skim or 1 percent milk
1 cup of fat-free or low-fat yogurt
$1^1/_2$ ounces of low-fat natural cheese

Protein Group (calories vary)
3 ounces of cooked lean meat, poultry, or fish (equal in size to a
    deck of playing cards)
    Women should limit their daily intake to 6 ounces (two decks);
        men can aim for 6 to 9 ounces daily (two to three decks)
$^1/_2$ cup of cooked beans
1 egg (yolk and white)
2 egg whites
2 tablespoons of natural peanut butter

MORE GOOD PROTEIN IS NOT BETTER

Although fish and poultry contain fewer calories and saturated fat per ounce than red meat, that doesn't mean you can eat larger portions of them. Portions of any type of meat should be about 3 to 4.5 ounces, the size of one to one and a half decks of playing cards. To understand how eating large portions of healthy protein may affect weight loss, consider these two scenarios.

HAMBURGER	HADDOCK
3 ounces	6 ounces
90 calories/ounce	55 calories/ounce
Calories consumed: 270	Calories consumed: 330

For weight loss, it would be better to eat a small hamburger than a large piece of haddock, which is a low-fat fish. If you substituted a fatty fish, the calories would go up even higher (closer to 500 calories for a 6-ounce piece of salmon).

Be smart about your sweet tooth: You don't have to give up sweets completely, but you will have to cultivate discipline. Limit consumption of sweets to one dessert a day or less. Although many people worry that desserts are diet busters, it doesn't have to be that way. To gain one pound of fat, you have to consume 3,500 additional calories. Eating the occasional piece of chocolate cake, at 350 calories, delivers only one-tenth of that amount. (It's habitual intake, day after day, and multiple daily servings that wreak havoc with your weight.) To stay on the safe side, restrict consumption of sweets to 200 calories a day or less, about the amount you'd find in one cup of low-fat frozen yogurt or four Fig Newton cookies.

Don't be fooled into thinking you can eat larger portions of low-fat desserts, though, because these are often loaded with sugar and have as many calories per serving as desserts that are high in fat. (The same is true for items like baked tortilla chips, which have about the same number of calories per chip as fried tortilla chips.) Eat too many of these "low-fat" alternatives, and you'll consume extra calories that are converted into—you guessed it— body fat. To limit portion sizes of items like ice cream, use cones (which hold less than a bowl) or teacups. You can also choose fruit instead of cookies or pastry and obtain an added bonus in the form of fiber, nutrients, and phytochemicals.

Beware of hidden fats: Sometimes we end up killing ourselves with the best of intentions. Choose a mixed green salad for lunch, and then drown it in salad dressing, and you may end up ingesting more calories than if you had eaten a hamburger. Hidden fats are everywhere: in baked goods and condiments like sour cream, cream cheese, salad dressing, and mayonnaise. They can also lurk in seemingly healthy choices in restaurants, such as Caesar salad and tuna fish salad sandwiches (often the selections with most calories because they are smothered in dressing and mayonnaise). Choose light or low-fat condiments, dressings, and sauces, and you will save calories as long as you watch the serving size. (Substituting one tablespoon of reduced-fat mayonnaise for the regular kind will save you 50 calories. Substitute a tablespoon of nonfat plain yogurt for the same amount of regular mayonnaise and you save 93 calories.) If you purchase full-fat varieties of these food add-ons, measure and limit your servings. And whenever possible, choose foods and condiments with healthy unsaturated fat over those with unhealthy saturated and trans fats.

■ Become a Mindful Eater

Can you remember whether or not you enjoyed your last meal? How long did it take you to eat the meal? Did you realize if you were full or not? What are some adjectives to describe the food in your mouth as you ate it? The answers to these questions indicate whether you are a mindless eater or a mindful eater.

If you have a hard time remembering what you ate last, never mind what it tasted and felt like, you are not alone. Americans often eat while doing other things. In this era of multitasking, one thing that gets shoved aside is mealtime. Lunch becomes just another annoyance that takes time away from more important tasks, rather than being viewed as a welcome and enjoyable break.

It doesn't have to be that way. If you set aside time to eat, without being distracted by other activities, you will find that you eat less but enjoy your food more.

To become a mindful eater, separate eating from your other activities. Mealtime should be a pleasurable experience, one that ideally involves sufficient time and a nice setting. Benefits of mindful eating include:

1. You will eat less food.
2. You will become more aware of feeling satisfied and avoid negative feelings caused by overeating and indigestion.
3. You will be able to indulge in an occasional moderate portion of a high-calorie food.
4. Your digestion will improve, because you will chew your food more thoroughly.
5. You will taste and enjoy what you eat.

One important aspect of becoming mindful about any experience is to slow down so that you notice the details. To become a mindful eater, try to take at least twenty minutes to eat a meal. This allows you to appreciate the flavor and texture of the food in your mouth. If you eat too quickly, you don't give your stomach time to fill sufficiently and send chemical signals to your brain indicating that you are satiated.

Try this informal assignment: Eat a meal or snack as slowly as possible. Pay attention to the tastes and textures that you are experiencing. Savor the food so that you really appreciate the flavors and experience the enjoyment of eating. Now think about what you noticed. How did the food taste? (Sweet? Salty? Tart?) How did it feel on your tongue? (Coarse? Smooth? A little of both?) Did you chew slowly so that you could taste the food before swallowing? Did you absorb the aroma before putting the food in your mouth? How long did it take you to eat the food?

■ Recognize Food Triggers

Beyond being mindful of what you're eating and how much, it also helps to become mindful of *why* you're eating. Are you really hungry? Or are some other cues triggering your eating behavior?

Remove temptations to prevent cravings: Many people tend to overeat simply because food is readily available. Think about the last time you attended a buffet brunch or dined at a restaurant with an all-you-can-eat policy. Did you heap too much food on your plate just because it was available, free, and tempting? Of course, if you do this only on occasion, it is probably not a problem. But what about for those who are constantly faced with food everywhere, at every time? Is your freezer stocked with your favorite ice cream? Do you have coworkers who keep candy in jars on their desks? To pass up these kinds of temptations requires remarkable willpower.

To eat healthfully and avoid weight gain, remove the temptations from your work and home environments. Throw or give the problematic food away. Don't rationalize that you are keeping cookies and candy around "for the children, grandchildren, or unexpected guests." If the food is there for others, then you may be tempted to think, "I can pass it up if I want to" or "I can eat just one." The truth is, most people can't.

Something else to consider: Why feed your family and friends the very food that you are trying to avoid? This is especially true when it comes to your children and grandchildren. Dietary habits begin early in life, and so do weight problems. In the United States in the last two decades, the number of children ages six to eleven who are overweight has doubled and the number of overweight adolescents (ages twelve to nineteen) has tripled. About one in ten children and adolescents in this country is considered seriously overweight. Don't let your child (or grandchild) be one of them.

Recognize emotional eating: Emotions can also trigger food cravings. Have you ever had a bad day and decided you needed a treat? Or celebrated something good with food? One patient who participated in our Cardiac Wellness Program got everyone laughing and nodding in agreement when she described her relationship with food. We'll call her Joanne. "When my husband lost his job, I ate a whole box of cookies in one sitting," Joanne told us. "When my son came home and told me he was getting married, I cooked a big dinner to celebrate. When my mother became seriously ill, I eased the ache I felt inside by filling my stomach with anything I could get my hands on. No matter what life handed me, good or bad, food got me through it."

Loneliness, frustration, boredom, anger, and depression can all trigger an eating binge. Food provides a quick fix; it is readily available, comforting, and feels good—at least in the short term. The problem, of course, is that over the long term, the effects of overeating do not feel good. Using food to improve mood leads into a vicious downward cycle: "I eat when I'm depressed, and then I feel guilty about my lack of self-control and how I look, so I eat some more to feel better."

When you find yourself reaching for food because you feel bad, remember the same strategy we discussed in Chapter 4 for stress control:

1. Stop (Stop yourself before eating food automatically.)
2. Breathe (This will not only relax you but will also prevent you from eating automatically.)
3. Reflect (Why do you want to eat at this moment? Is it hunger or because you feel depressed, anxious, stressed, or bored?)
4. Choose (If you are eating because of a negative emotion, not hunger, you can choose a nonfood-related activity to make yourself feel better. See our suggestions in Sidebar 36, page 203.)

This four-step strategy helps to reduce impulse eating because it gives you time to think and make a different choice. If you don't stop to think about what is going on, then you will react in a knee-jerk fashion and will likely eat 100 percent of the time. By stopping yourself and taking time to breathe, reflect, and choose, you will prevent yourself from bingeing at least some of the time.

To put this into practice, think about what nonfood activities improve your mood. Write them down and place the list on your refrigerator or on the back of the cookie cupboard door. Identify some specific activities that you can use the next time you feel bad and want to eat. If you truly are hungry, choose a healthy snack, a small portion of a high-calorie food, and eat it mindfully, or drink a calorie-free beverage.

Manage your overeating chain: The overeating chain is a sequence of actions and feelings that ends in dietary disaster. One action naturally leads to the next, and you end up eating too much and then feeling bad about it. In describing this sort of behavior, people are not usually aware of the events that take place before they overeat. As one of our patients once put it, "I eat a big bowl of ice cream every night; I don't know why I do it. I know it isn't good for me to eat ice cream so often, but I seem to have no willpower in the evening."

As you can see in the diagram in Table 19, page 204, though, a

---

NO-CALORIE ALTERNATIVES

Many of these suggestions work because they are pleasurable and boost your mood. Others (such as cleaning the house) may distract you long enough so that you can outlast a craving.

Mood Boosters and Distractions

Take a shower or bubble bath.

Take a walk.

Elicit the relaxation response.

Spend time with family members.

Spend time with a pet.

Call a friend.

Clean the house.

Do a hobby (crossword puzzle, carpentry, knitting, quilting.)

Shop for clothing.

Treat yourself to a facial, pedicure, or manicure.

---

series of individual events led to that big bowl of ice cream. Fortunately, it is possible to break the overeating chain anywhere along the continuum. Since a lot of people overeat while watching television, one strategy is to use time after dinner to engage in another activity, such as taking a walk, making telephone calls, or playing with children or a pet. Or break the chain further into the evening: Decide ahead of time that if you get bored while watching television, you will read a novel, not walk into the kitchen. (Place the book on a table near the TV to firm up your resolve.) Or break the chain even later by having a scheduled evening snack, but by making it a low-calorie one (one cup of low-fat frozen yogurt or fresh fruit, for instance).

It may help to map out your own overeating chain, especially if you consistently overeat at the same time of day. That's a good indication that your overeating behavior follows a predictable pattern. Think of ways to break the chain at various links by

---

TABLE 19

THE OVEREATING CHAIN

After dinner, sit in favorite chair.

↓

Watch TV.

↓

Feel bored.

↓

Go to kitchen.

↓

Look for food.

↓

Eat large bowl of premium ice cream.

↓

Feel bad about self.

---

changing your routine, and that will stop the triggers. We can't guarantee that you can always prevent yourself from overeating, but every time you manage to avoid it you help your heart.

■ Mind over Matter: Losing Weight

If you are overweight or obese, you will do your heart a lot of good if you shed pounds. Losing weight helps to lower blood pressure and improve cholesterol levels in overweight people, while reducing blood sugar levels.

That doesn't mean that you have to starve yourself back to your high school or military weight, though. Many people have unrealistic expectations for how much they can—or should—lose. One study found that people on a diet intended to lose 30 percent of their body weight. Not surprisingly, most of them failed to come even close to meeting this goal. Any weight reduction will help improve your heart health, so every pound lost is a step in the right direction.

One note of caution: If you have quit smoking in the past six months, defer any attempt at weight loss and concentrate instead on maintaining your current weight. Staying away from cigarettes will do more for your health than losing weight. Physical activity helps in this regard: Studies show that people who quit smoking and are able to best maintain a healthy weight are those who exercise regularly.

Set realistic goals: If you're thinking about losing weight, choose a goal that is realistic and achievable. The latest research indicates that you can reasonably aim to reduce your weight by 10 percent over six months, and then maintain the new weight before attempting to lose anymore. (So if you weigh 180 pounds, losing 18 pounds is reasonable.)

Plan for a slow burn: Crash dieting, either by skipping meals or drastically reducing your calorie intake, is one of the worst things you can do when trying to lose weight. People who crash diet and initially lose a large amount of weight are losing mostly fluid and muscle tissue and tend to gain weight back very quickly. Crash dieting also wreaks havoc with your resting metabolic rate—the rate at which calories are burned to keep the body functioning. Confronted with a sudden and severe reduction in calories, your body reacts as if you were starving and begins to conserve energy.

Metabolism slows significantly—by as much as 45 percent—so that you lose no additional weight despite reducing calorie intake.

A slow, steady weight loss is better. People who lose a half pound to two pounds per week are more likely to develop good long-term eating habits, lose a greater percentage of the weight as fat, and maintain fat loss over the long term. To prevent your resting metabolism from dropping as you diet, eat at regular intervals throughout the day but reduce portions and calories. Exercise regularly, which helps to prevent your resting metabolism from dropping and improves your ability to burn calories. (More on this in Chapter 8.)

Reduce total calories: Many people focus only on reducing fat as they try to lose weight, and may fall into the common trap of believing that "fat-free" foods and snacks can be consumed without worry. This is not true, as all foods have some calories (see Sidebar 37, below). Your body can turn any excess calories into fat, so pay attention to total calories consumed. To reduce calories without feeling hungry all the time, we recommend the following:

1. Balance your plate at every meal, even snacks. Always include a source of protein or healthy fat to make you feel full. Avoid meals and snacks consisting only of carbohydrates because you won't feel satisfied and may overeat and want to eat again sooner than usual.

SIDEBAR 37

CALORIES COMPARED

Fat	9 calories/gram
Alcohol	7 calories/gram
Carbohydrates	4 calories/gram
Protein	4 calories/gram

---

2. Pay special attention to portion sizes. Some people find it helpful to use measuring cups when adding to their plate, to prevent overdoing it.

Watch liquid calories: Reduce consumption of sugared soft drinks and alcohol, or avoid these beverages altogether. Limit consumption of fruit juice, which is healthy but also high in calories. One 6-ounce glass of fruit juice a day is sufficient; if you love the taste and want more, dilute the juice with water or seltzer water so that you don't add calories. Often people forget about how many calories they ingest each day in liquid form. (Several studies even suggest that drinking high-calorie beverages may actually prompt you to consume *more* food at a meal.) A regular beer (12 ounces) contains 150 calories, 4 ounces of dry wine has 80 calories, and a 2½-ounce martini has 156 calories. Drink just one can of regular beer or a sugared soda per day, without decreasing consumption of other calories or increasing activity, and you could gain fifteen pounds by the end of the year. To cut down on liquid calories, choose water, flavored seltzer water, sugar-free soft drinks on occasion, and light beer. If you prefer wine, try a wine spritzer, which is half wine, half seltzer water and cuts the calories in half. When you go out socially, try alternating alcoholic with low-calorie nonalcoholic beverages.

Reduce saturated and trans fat intake: Since fats are the most concentrated sources of calories in your diet, lowering daily intake of unhealthy fats will help you to lose weight. The challenge is to maintain consumption of the healthy ones. (For more information, see pages 158 to 164 in Chapter 6.)

Use sugar sparingly: White sugar is fine, as long as you limit consumption to a few teaspoons a day. (Contrary to popular belief, honey and brown sugar are not nutritionally superior to sugar. Natural molasses—not the sugary alternatives found in many stores—is the sole exception. It is a good source of iron, calcium, and potassium.) We don't recommend that you replace your table sugar with sugar substitutes such as Equal or NutraSweet. A teaspoon of table sugar contains only 15 calories and 4 grams of sugar, which is not a lot to begin with. In addition, sugar substitutes have certainly done nothing to stem the obesity epidemic in this country. Rather than focusing on reducing your consumption of table sugar, consume fewer soft drinks, juices, and desserts (even the low-fat kind), since they contain a large amount of sugar.

If you lapse, try again: If you lapse and go off your diet, don't compound the problem by beating yourself up. Figure out what caused you to overeat and see if you can avoid it in the future. As the great Chinese philosopher Confucius put it, "Our greatest glory is not in never failing, but in rising every time we fall."

Journalist Anne Fletcher interviewed about two hundred people for her book *Thin for Life*. Most of the people she interviewed tried five to six diets before finally losing weight. Although following a low-calorie diet was clearly important, so was cultivating particular mental "attitudes," such as optimism, positive reinforcement, and a sense of social support. Use lapses as learning experiences for the future rather than as reasons to call yourself a failure. (For more advice on dealing with relapses, see Chapter 9.)

Keep moving: Physical activity is essential for any weight loss program because it increases the number of calories you burn per day, keeps your metabolism revved up, and helps increase muscle mass (which consumes more calories than fat). Small wonder, studies have shown, that people who exercise regularly are best able to lose weight and keep it off. Choose something that you enjoy and will fit into your normal routine. See Chapter 8 for more information on how to build exercise into your life.

Chapter 8

Exercise Body and Soul

If exercise could be put in a pill, it would be the most widely prescribed medicine in the world.
— DR. ROBERT N. BUTLER, NATIONAL INSTITUTE ON AGING

M ENTION PHYSICAL ACTIVITY, and many people immediately think of something negative: the gym class they dreaded in seventh grade, the ache of tired muscles, the fear of not being good enough. Even though most people know about the health benefits of exercise, they view it as something they *have* to do because it is good for them. It's like taking a medication. No wonder people have a hard time getting motivated.

In this chapter, we hope to convince you that exercise is a gift— not a burden. We want it to become something you *want* to do, rather than something you *have* to do. Physical activity will then become part of who you are. It will become a treasured "time-out" from the demands of the day, one that you can't imagine doing without.

How does this attitude shift take place? One important step is to learn to regard physical activity as a way of reinvigorating your mind as well as your body. In our Cardiac Wellness Program, we offer a holistic approach to exercise that is based on the premise that mind and body are not separate but, instead, different expressions of our fundamental life force.

Our holistic mind/body approach involves three key elements.

THE GIFT OF EXERCISE

The other day, I was looking for a gift to give to a friend. This friend is very important to me and I want her to be around for a long time. I want her to live a long and healthy life. I thought how great it would be if I could give her a gift that would improve the quality of her life.

So I sat down and made a list of what I would look for in this special gift:

- It would help her to be stronger, firmer, leaner, more flexible, and energetic.
- It would help lower her risk of dying from heart disease, help lower blood pressure and improve lipid profile, control blood glucose level, and fight obesity.
- It would help maintain balance and bone density, and help her age more gracefully.
- It would help improve immune system function, concentration, task performance, and quality of sleep.
- It would help reduce stress, improve mood, enhance self-esteem, and increase optimism and confidence.
- It would help increase self-awareness, spiritual well-being, and control over choices in her life.
- It would be fun but also challenging.
- It would allow for socialization but also for time alone, depending on her needs.
- It would come in all different modes and styles and could be adapted to various environments and weather conditions.
- Finally, it would have a good *Consumer Reports* rating, supported by scientific data from reputable sources.

After completing my list, I realized that the only gift that meets all my criteria is the gift of exercise. Have a healthy and happy life, my friend.

—*Jim Huddleston, M.S., P.T., Cardiac Wellness Program*

Two—cardiovascular activities for endurance and musculoskeletal exercises for strength and flexibility—will sound familiar. The third element, body awareness, makes our program unique. Body awareness involves paying attention to what you are feeling while you exercise: What feels good and what does not? If you learn to

---

TABLE 20

THE ELEMENTS OF HOLISTIC EXERCISE

A mind/body approach to exercise encompasses the traditional elements of exercise but also adds an element: body awareness. This approach requires adopting a different mind-set toward exercise than you may be used to.

Type of Exercise	Traditional View	Holistic Mind/Body View
Aerobic exercise (Examples: walking, swimming, bicycling)	• Improves cardiovascular fitness • Increases endurance • Enables physical activity for extended periods without fatigue	• Focus is internal • Focus on breath rhythm and deep abdominal breathing • Focus on cadence of steps while walking or jogging, on pedaling while riding a bicycle, or on arm strokes while swimming
Musculoskeletal exercises (Examples: lifting weights, muscle stretches)	• Increases muscle strength • Increases overall flexibility • Reduces risk for injury during normal daily tasks	• Movements slow and rhythmic, coordinated with breathing • Focus is internal: how the muscles feel as they move • Uses yoga to realign posture, release tension, and maintain a basic "resting state" • Uses Tai Chi as a "moving meditation" to provide focus for the body and mind

(continued on next page)

Type of Exercise	Traditional View	Holistic Mind/Body View
Body awareness	Not part of the traditional view	• Focus is on listening to the messages from your body rather than trying to meet an external goal (such as number of minutes or calories burned) • Make decisions about how long or how hard to exercise based on feedback from your body • Facilitates self-knowledge and acceptance • Relieves stress and reduces risk for injury

listen to your body and respond to how you feel, you will know when to ease off and take it easy and when to push a little harder. You will learn to listen to messages from your body as you move and to make choices based on what you "hear." This approach to exercise not only tunes your body, it also facilitates self-acceptance and self-knowledge. As physician and runner George Sheehan once wrote, "The body mirrors the mind and soul and is much more accessible than either. If you can become proficient at listening to your body, you will eventually hear from your whole self." In the long term this attitude helps you mentally as well as physically.

In this way, exercise becomes a means of self-observation, a way to increase self-awareness, rather than just an outcome-oriented activity with a physical focus. When you begin to view exercise as a way of life and not as an obligation, then you are truly on the path to improving your physical and spiritual health.

▦ Learning from Other Cultures

When it comes to broadening our perspective about exercise, we have much to learn from other cultures. In our goal-oriented Western culture, exercise is measured by minutes, calories, and pain. Often lost in the process is any sense of enjoyment.

Other cultures provide a different perspective and may suggest ways to broaden your own thinking. In ancient traditions, physical activity and exercise had less of a physical focus and more of a spiritual one. The Greek philosopher Plato, for instance, regarded exercise as a means of developing one's spiritual life. He viewed exercise as a way to attain the harmonious perfection of body, mind, and soul. According to the Vedic text of Buddhism, the main purpose of exercise is to rejuvenate the body and cultivate the mind, developing coordination between the two.

Even today, many cultures use physical activity as a way to celebrate history and community. In Africa, for instance, dance is often used to celebrate life, culture, and generate healing. In the African healing dances, dancers mimic the movements of animals and nature to connect with the world and draw healing energy from it. Similarly, Native American people in this country have long used dances for ceremony, storytelling, and entertainment— not just exercise. The hoop dance, which honors the unbroken circle of life, is just one example.

Yoga, which originated in India but has become very popular in the United States, is as much a philosophy as it is a physical practice. The word *yoga* means "union" or "joining together." True to its name, yoga is a type of exercise that enables you to develop and maintain musculoskeletal health by realigning your posture, releasing tension, and increasing flexibility, while also helping to cultivate mind/body awareness. These are some reasons we recommend yoga as one way to elicit the relaxation response. (See Chapter 3.)

Another Eastern exercise practice, Tai Chi, which originated in

China, combines movement with focused awareness in order to enable a life force known as *qi* to flow through the body. Tai Chi is known as a "moving meditation," and if you've seen it done, you know why: Practitioners move slowly and fluidly, as if dancing in slow motion. These graceful exercises relieve tension, improve balance and coordination, foster strength and flexibility, and focus the mind. (For a sample Tai Chi practice, see page 252.)

■ The Benefits of Exercise

We are born to move. To remain healthy, we need to remain physically active. Regular exercise not only provides a number of overall health benefits, but it is particularly beneficial to the heart.

You might say it's been hardwired into us. Centuries ago, physical fitness helped our ancestors survive as hunters and farmers, especially when living conditions were especially harsh. Only quite recently, in evolutionary terms, has technology freed us from the need to be active in order to survive. Machines and computers now do much of our work. Automobiles, buses, and trains enable us to get from one place to another without walking. Escalators and elevators climb for us. Television provides entertainment and demands nothing more than that we sit on the couch. With remote controls, we do not even have to get up to change channels. Small wonder that Americans have become so sedentary.

Although some experts advise doing more activity, we follow the guidelines issued in a 2001 report by the U.S. Surgeon General, which recommended that people exercise thirty minutes a day, most days a week, aiming for three to four hours a week. This physical activity does not have to be extremely vigorous, as we will discuss below. Yet the Surgeon General estimated that fewer than one in three Americans engage in the minimum amount of physical activity recommended by the federal government. And four in ten American adults participate in no physical activity during their leisure time. Other studies have shown that only 20 to 25 percent of Americans—fewer than one in four—exercise enough to obtain any significant health benefits, and fewer than one in ten exercise at the intensity required for improving cardiovascular health.

A sedentary lifestyle can be deadly. More than one in ten deaths in this country—250,000 per year—are related to lack of regular physical activity. Among other things, a sedentary lifestyle increases the risk for overweight and obesity, diabetes, high blood pressure, and potentially life-threatening arrhythmias. On the other hand, more than thirty years of research shows that regular exercise promotes physical and psychological health in a wide variety of ways. Physical activity helps our bodies function more efficiently, burn calories supplied by food, and use fat stores as a fuel source (thus helping us lose weight). Moreover, exercise tones muscles, strengthens bones, and improves endurance, stamina, and mood.

Regular physical activity also increases our chances of living longer. One research study conducted over a five-year period found that previously sedentary men who became physically fit were 44 percent less likely to die during that time (and 52 percent less likely to suffer from cardiovascular disease) than men who remained unfit. Other studies suggest that physically active people tend to live one to two years longer than their sedentary peers. That may not seem significant, but the real gain comes in terms of functional independence. Regular physical activity slows the deterioration associated with the so-called normal aging process (which may not be so normal at all), such as loss of muscle strength, bone mass, and impairments in sleep, sex, and cognitive function. There are even several cancers that occur less often in people who exercise regularly. "Good nutrition and regular exercise do reduce the risk of various diseases . . . thereby serving as the best current prescription for a long and healthy life," write three experts on aging, S. Jay Olshansky, Leonard Hayflick, and Bruce Carnes.

It's a common belief that the main benefit from exercise is weight loss. Therefore, some people figure that if they are not overweight, they don't stand to benefit from exercise. That is wrong. All the benefits of exercise apply just as much for people of normal weight.

■ Exercise Is Good for Your Heart

Physical activity is particularly beneficial for your heart. It not only helps to prevent heart disease but also improves your chances of recovery and survival if you have already suffered a heart attack or some other type of coronary event.

Several studies suggest that the more physically fit you are, the lower your chances are of developing heart disease or suffering a heart attack. People who exercise regularly, for instance, are less likely to suffer a heart attack during heavy physical exertion, a well-known trigger of a coronary event. In fact, a recent study found that low exercise capacity may be as powerful a predictor of mortality as other cardiac risk factors such as hypertension, smoking, and diabetes. Sedentary living increases risk for heart disease almost as much as other factors such as high blood pressure, elevated cholesterol, and cigarette smoking. The evidence is so compelling, in fact, that physical inactivity is now recognized as one of the four major risk factors for heart disease. (See Chapter 2.)

Sedentary living not only presents a risk in its own right; it can also worsen the effects of other risk factors. The flip side of this coin is that if you become physically active you can help to counteract the adverse effects of other risk factors such as high blood pressure, high cholesterol, and obesity. One study involving a group of men at high risk for heart attack and sudden death demonstrated this conclusion dramatically. All the men smoked and had either high blood pressure or high cholesterol or both. Those who were moderately active were only 63 percent as likely to suffer from coronary heart disease or experience sudden death from a heart attack as the least active men. Another study concluded that men and women with multiple risk factors for heart disease but who were physically fit were less likely to die than out-of-shape people with no risk factors.

How does exercise work its magic on the heart? A number of physiological and metabolic mechanisms are at work.

Improves lipid profile: Exercise affects the metabolism of cholesterol and thereby improves your overall lipid profile. Various studies show that exercise increases helpful HDL cholesterol, while lowering levels of potentially harmful triglycerides. But exercise is not a quick fix. In order for exercise to benefit your cholesterol levels, you need to be active on a regular basis and make it a lifetime habit.

Lowers blood pressure: People who are inactive and not physically fit are also about 30 to 50 percent more likely to develop high blood pressure than those who do get regular physical activity. When you do aerobic exercise such as taking a walk or riding a bicycle, arteries throughout your body widen to accommodate an increase in blood flow, and pressure on the arterial walls decreases. Scientists speculate that the repetitive widening and narrowing of artery walls helps maintain vascular elasticity and helps maintain normal blood pressure. It may take a few months to notice significant results from exercise, so don't get discouraged. The wait may well be worth it: In some people, low- to moderate-intensity exercise may be as effective as medication in lowering blood pressure.

Helps maintain healthy weight: People who are obese are at greater risk for heart disease than their leaner peers, and exercise clearly plays a role in maintaining a healthy weight. Physical activity helps you burn calories throughout the day, not just while you are active, and a healthy diet decreases the number of calories you ingest. (See Chapter 7.) We'll discuss ways to use exercise to lose weight later in this chapter. (See page 239).

Reduces risk of developing diabetes: Exercise combined with a healthy diet can help to prevent the development of non-insulin dependent diabetes (the most common kind) and the concomitant risk to your heart. Although we are still trying to understand all the mechanisms involved, it appears that exercise counters insulin resistance by increasing sensitivity to this hormone and enhancing its effect in the body. Exercise also reduces the risk for obesity, which contributes to the development of diabetes. With the right combination of diet and exercise, many people with non-insulin dependent diabetes can avoid having to take glucose-lowering medications and yet still maintain normal blood sugar levels. (For special exercise tips for people with diabetes, see page 243).

Reduces risk for blood clots: Regular exercise reduces the risk that you will develop a blood clot that can lead to a heart attack. Although more research is needed before we fully understand why this is so, it appears that regular physical activity enhances the effects of natural anticlotting chemicals in the blood and prevents blood platelets from sticking together.

Reduces risk for arrhythmia: Regular physical activity reduces the heart's sensitivity to catecholamines, hormones released as part of the stress response, which can cause irregular—and sometimes fatal—heartbeats known as ventricular arrhythmias.

Counters psychological risks: Exercise also helps the heart by counteracting many of the psychological factors that contribute to heart disease. A number of studies show, for instance, that regular physical activity will lessen feelings of depression and anxiety while bolstering an overall sense of well-being. A team led by James Blumenthal at Duke University Medical Center even found that regular aerobic exercise could be as effective as an antidepressant in reducing symptoms of depression in older individuals. In a follow-up study ten months later, Blumenthal's team found that people who still exercised not only continued to benefit but were also less likely than those on medication to suffer a relapse of depressive symptoms.

Other studies have shown that exercise reduces elements of type A behavior that are toxic to the heart, while improving physical, psychological, and even social well-being. Exercise also helps people withstand the effects of stress, possibly by reducing physical strain on the body and by increasing stress hardiness. Studies suggest further that the more physically active you are, the better you feel.

■ Exercise Is Good for Your Body

Although the focus of this book is heart health, regular physical activity provides additional benefits that motivate many people to get off the couch and start moving.

Exercise helps you look better: Regular physical activity, done over a prolonged period, will reshape your body. Exercise builds muscle and burns fat—both the fat located under the skin (where you may be able to pinch more than an inch of flesh) and that contained within the muscle itself. The more muscle you have, the more calories you burn all day long—so lowering your percentage of body fat while increasing muscle is an investment that "pays off" throughout the day. The combination of exercise and a healthy diet is the only successful long-term weight loss and maintenance program.

Exercise helps you do better: Various studies have shown that much of the physical deterioration that takes place between ages thirty and seventy is related to sedentary lifestyle, not advancing age. One study found, for instance, that a thirty-year-old man who remains moderately active and maintains relatively low body fat will lose only half as much of his aerobic capacity as may be expected by age seventy. Studies in women have provided similar findings. Aerobic capacity is important because it reflects the ability of your cardiovascular system to deliver and use oxygen, which in turn affects endurance and ability to function and live independently.

Exercise is also vital to musculoskeletal health. Movement places mechanical stress on bones, cartilage, and muscle, which helps to circulate nutrients and stimulate natural self-repair mechanisms. Exercise appears to minimize bone loss that can occur with age and encourage new bone growth. Exercise helps joints by moving them on a regular basis. The pressure of movement bathes joints in the nutrient-rich lubricant that surrounds them, known as synovial fluid. Muscles grow lean and strong with use, especially when challenged by resistance exercises.

Good musculoskeletal health (along with cardiovascular fitness) helps to explain why physically active people can expect to enjoy an extra ten to twenty years of living independently. So "use it or lose it" is a good philosophy. And no matter how old you are, it's never too late to start. Studies demonstrate that even eighty- and ninety-year-old people have the ability to increase muscle strength, walking speed, and ability to climb stairs—all skills that enable them to live more independently.

Exercise helps you feel better: We've already discussed the positive impact exercise has on mood. In addition, exercise will help you feel more energetic and less susceptible to fatigue—partly because your endurance will increase and partly because you will sleep better. You will not feel better overnight, of course, because the benefits increase with time. But they will be real—and striking. In fact, a number of epidemiological studies found that exercise has a significant impact on immune function. An example is the relationship between exercise and upper respiratory tract infections (such as colds and flu). While sedentary people appear to have an average risk for upper respiratory tract infections, moderate exercise (i.e., brisk walking) decreases the risk.

Although we are still trying to determine all the ways that exercise affects immune system function, it is clear that people who exercise on a regular basis don't become ill as often as sedentary people do. It appears that moderate physical activity triggers the release of hormones that stimulate the immune system, which, in turn, increases the number and activity of certain protective cells.

▉ Exercise Is Good for Your Soul

We are made of more than just cells and chemicals, of course. Physical activity also provides a way to get in touch with your innermost self: your spirit, your soul. This is especially true when exercise is combined with the relaxation response, which we explored in detail in Chapter 3. When you use exercise to elicit the relaxation response, the result is a tremendous release of tension and, in its place, an enhanced feeling of well-being. Exercising in this way helps you learn more about yourself. You will exercise your spirit as well as your body.

The key to developing this approach to exercise is to shift your focus away from goals (number of calories burned, number of minutes spent exercising) and instead focus on the process: how you feel as you move. To help maintain an in-tune state of mind, it is helpful to employ the two components central to eliciting the relaxation response—a repetitive focus, or mechanism (breath rhythm, a mantra, or a physical rhythm) and a nonjudging attitude (accepting the experience as it happens) toward your activity.

To exercise your soul by eliciting the relaxation response, any physical activity will do as long as it fits the following descriptors:

- Enjoyable (facilitates a relaxed attitude)
- Noncompetitive (competition implies judgment)
- Predictable (provides a sense of safety and reliability)
- Repetitive and rhythmic (provides a focus for awareness)
- Involves abdominal breathing (the key to relaxation)
- Lasts for twenty to thirty minutes (facilitates a conditioning effect for mindful exercise)

Many yoga postures embody these characteristics; so does swimming or taking a walk. Aerobic exercise is particularly useful in eliciting the relaxation response, since it involves deep breathing and a particular rhythm. In whatever way you choose to elicit the relaxation response, remember to adopt a nonjudging attitude and an inward focus as you do it. You'll soon discover your spirit! Exercise for fitness of the spirit and soul and just let your body do the work.

One example of how to exercise your soul as well as your body is to "enlighten the dumbbells," which we'll describe next (see Sidebar 39, page 223). You'll find other suggestions at the end of the chapter, where we'll discuss Tai Chi and mindful walking.

■ Your Exercise Prescription

How much exercise do you need and what kind should you do in order to gain all the benefits you can? The federal government has established minimum guidelines for how much physical activity is needed to enhance your health, based on a number of studies, which we'll discuss in the pages that follow. These detailed recommendations on how much to exercise may seem at first to contradict our earlier advice of "letting go" of goals. Our philosophy however, adapts quite simply: Know what you're aiming for, but remember that something is better than nothing. All too often, people who have led mainly sedentary lives are intimidated by the thought of suddenly committing themselves to an exercise regimen. So whatever you do, start slowly and build gradually, over a matter of weeks or even months, if that's what it takes.

■ Building a Fitness Foundation

In the 1970s and 1980s, "no pain, no gain" was the common mantra. The recommendations by the government, media, and private trainers for exercise were so demanding that many Americans couldn't meet them, got discouraged, and gave up. Hoping to encourage people to get off the couch, scientists from the Centers for Disease Control and Prevention and the American College of Sports Medicine convened a panel in the mid-1990s to review the body of evidence on exercise. They concluded that moderate

---

SIDEBAR 39

ENLIGHTENING THE DUMBBELLS

The next time you lift weights, try this approach and see if you feel reinvigorated spiritually afterward:

- Focus on your breath, your form, the sensation of your muscles lifting the weight.
- Move the weight slowly along with the rhythm of your breath; breathe out as you lift the weight, breathe in as you return to the starting position.
- Pay attention to how your body feels, not to your mind telling you to hurry up or lift more weight.
- When you do increase the amount of weight you lift, watch your form to avoid injury.
- Let go of distracting thoughts and bring awareness back to the breath.

---

exercise offered people the most overall health benefits and that it was the number of calories expended on exercise each week—not the intensity, length, or type of activity—that really mattered. As a result, the scientists issued a new set of guidelines that can be summarized by the phrase "less pain, more gain."

Follow these recommendations, and you will be well on your way to building a foundation for fitness:

SIDEBAR 40

WHEN TO SEE A DOCTOR

Many people can begin to engage in moderate physical activity without worry, but if you have either heart disease, two or more of the risk factors listed below, or a pulmonary or metabolic disease, consult your doctor before starting a new exercise program.

Age Precautions:

- Men older than 40
- Women older than 50

Coronary Risk Factors:

- High blood pressure
- Elevated cholesterol
- Cigarette smoking
- Abnormal resting EKG
- Family history of heart disease before age 50
- Diabetes

Metabolic Diseases:

- Thyroid disorders
- Renal (kidney) disease
- Liver disease

EXERCISE AFTER A CARDIAC EVENT

Most people who have had a heart attack, experienced angina, or undergone angioplasty can exercise safely. Indeed, your physician probably encourages you to become physically active and may have provided a referral to a cardiac rehabilitation program that includes exercise. Even so, if you have had a cardiac event, take a few extra precautions:

- Consult your physician before exercising, and ask if it is appropriate to undergo an exercise test (if you haven't already had one) to determine a safe level of activity.
- Ask your physician about specific activities you are interested in doing to determine if they are safe for you (i.e., lifting objects, shoveling snow, strenuous sports).
- Pay attention to the weather. Exercising when it is very hot or cold outside places additional demands on your heart.
- Stop exercising immediately if you experience:
  - Angina or increasing chest pain
  - Palpitations
  - Dizziness
  - Loss of muscle coordination
  - Severe fatigue
  - Shortness of breath
  - Wheezing
  - Leg cramps
- Reduce the intensity of your exercise if you experience:
  - Fatigue that lasts hours after finishing your activity
  - Muscle aches and pains that linger after exercise
- Listen to your body; don't push yourself too hard. Keep your efforts to a comfortable challenge.

- Accumulate thirty minutes or more of moderate-intensity physical activity on most (or all) days of the week; aim for three to four hours a week.
- The activity does not have to be continuous in order for you to obtain health benefits; ten-minute bouts of activity, done three times a day, are just as good as a continuous half-hour interval. To achieve enough exercise each day, you might do a brisk fifteen-minute walk before going to work, then park your car ten minutes away from your workplace and walk that distance briskly in the morning. By walking at a comparable pace back to your car at the end of the day, you compile thirty-five minutes of exercise. Be flexible so that you can make adjustments as needed. If it's going to rain today and tomorrow, think of an indoor location where you can walk during lunch or at the end of the day. (Malls can be good for this: They provide plenty of space and things to look at as you walk.) Or plan to walk for longer periods once the sun comes back out so that you still achieve your weekly goal. The bottom line is that you can organize the type of exercise you need into your life pretty easily.
- Exercising for 30 minutes will expend approximately 150 to 200 calories a day (the equivalent of walking two miles at a brisk pace). Doing this most days of the week will burn 1,000 to 1,400 calories a week—the figure that correlates with a gain in health benefits.
- Any activity is good if it gets you moving, but do a low-intensity activity for a longer period of time than you would one of high-intensity, since the benefits derive from the number of calories expended, not the number of minutes you stay active.
- Once you understand how to reach this goal, then you can let go of the numbers and simply enjoy the activity.

All sorts of activities count as you build your foundation of fitness: formal activities, such as an aerobics group or weight lifting

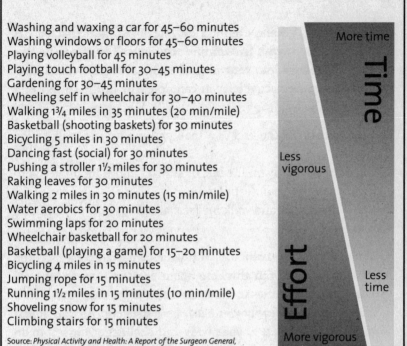

Washing and waxing a car for 45–60 minutes
Washing windows or floors for 45–60 minutes
Playing volleyball for 45 minutes
Playing touch football for 30–45 minutes
Gardening for 30–45 minutes
Wheeling self in wheelchair for 30–40 minutes
Walking 1¾ miles in 35 minutes (20 min/mile)
Basketball (shooting baskets) for 30 minutes
Bicycling 5 miles in 30 minutes
Dancing fast (social) for 30 minutes
Pushing a stroller 1½ miles for 30 minutes
Raking leaves for 30 minutes
Walking 2 miles in 30 minutes (15 min/mile)
Water aerobics for 30 minutes
Swimming laps for 20 minutes
Wheelchair basketball for 20 minutes
Basketball (playing a game) for 15–20 minutes
Bicycling 4 miles in 15 minutes
Jumping rope for 15 minutes
Running 1½ miles in 15 minutes (10 min/mile)
Shoveling snow for 15 minutes
Climbing stairs for 15 minutes

Source: *Physical Activity and Health: A Report of the Surgeon General,*
U.S. Department of Health and Human Services, 1996

Figure 24: How to burn about 150 calories

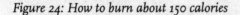

at a gym; informal activities, such as walking up the stairs rather than taking the elevator; recreational activities, such as tennis and golf (as long as you walk the fairways); even chores like housework or yard work. Remember, the more you do, the greater the health benefits you will enjoy. And those benefits don't level off until you burn several thousand calories a week—something few of us are in danger of doing.

■ Start Slowly and Persist

If the thought of doing even ten minutes of sustained activity is intimidating, start with five-minute segments. The way to do this is to build exercise into your normal daily activities. Some examples of five-minute activities you can do easily in the course of a day include the following:

- Park your car at the end of a mall parking lot and walk to the stores.
- Get off a stop early on the bus or subway and walk the remaining distance to your destination.
- Skip the elevator and walk up the stairs if it's only two or three flights.

You can probably come up with your own examples, too. The point is to expand your thinking about exercise, and to take advantage of opportunities to move throughout the day.

No matter how slowly you start, be persistent. As you adjust to more activity, listen to your body and challenge yourself to do better.

■ Improve Your Fitness Level

In addition to including physical activity in your everyday life, you can also start to improve your cardiovascular and musculoskeletal fitness. You don't have to add on a whole new exercise regimen. Instead, we suggest that you begin to pay more attention to the types of exercise you do, the amount of time you exercise each week, and how these choices fit into your life. For total fitness, aim to achieve a good balance between aerobic fitness, flexibility, and muscle toning.

Aerobic exercise: This type of activity raises heart rate and increases the rate of breathing, thereby stimulating the entire cardiovascular system. Examples include walking, swimming, bicycling, anything that is continuous and rhythmic and gets you breathing a little harder and your heart beating faster. Aerobic exercise takes energy; to supply it, your body uses oxygen to burn fat stores along with blood glucose to supply energy. Aerobic exercise is thus a wonderful way to maintain a healthy weight while also improving your endurance and the efficiency of your cardiovascular system.

What's the best aerobic exercise? The one you enjoy! With relative intensity being equal, the cardiovascular benefit of various aerobic activities is about the same. So pick the activity you enjoy most, because you will likely do that one on a regular basis. Walking is generally a good choice for most people. It doesn't require any special equipment or cost any money. You can do it alone or with friends, depending on your preference. And it travels well: You can walk while on vacation without having to pack it up and take it with you. A good goal is to aim to be physically active on most days for at least thirty minutes, but try not to miss more than two days in a row. The benefits of exercise are cumulative, and after forty-eight hours they begin to diminish.

If you have heart disease, and especially if you have already had a heart attack or some other type of cardiac event, check with your physician about what types of aerobic activities you can do safely. (See Sidebar 41, page 225.) Most people with heart disease can engage in any number of aerobic activities as long as they do them at moderate intensity. Remember, though, that physical activity does not take place in a vacuum. If you are feeling stress or exercising in extremely hot or cold weather, take special care not to overdo it.

If you have a musculoskeletal condition (such as arthritis), consider swimming, walking, or working out in a pool. You will weigh less underwater, and water provides support to your body, taking pressure off your bones and joints. Water also provides some resistance as you move through it, so it is a good environment for doing both weight training and aerobic exercise.

Muscle toning: This form of exercise, sometimes called resistance or weight training, is an example of anaerobic exercise. You engage in short bursts of activity, such as doing sit-ups or lifting weights, burning mostly blood sugar (glucose) to supply the energy needed for the activity. Activity happens too quickly to allow the body to use oxygen and burn fat for fuel. Muscle toning:

- Increases muscle strength/endurance
- Increases muscle mass
- Improves ability to burn calories; assists in weight loss
- Maintains or increases bone density
- Helps maintain the muscle strength necessary to perform everyday tasks

You can choose from different types of muscle toning devices and exercises, including:

- Free weights (including strap-on wrist and ankle weights)
- Weight machines (Nautilus, Universal, Cybex)
- Latex stretch bands
- Calisthenics (sit-ups, pull-ups, push-ups, press-ups)

We've included a few examples of exercises you can do at home to strengthen muscles in your upper and lower body; these can be combined with other exercises to achieve a total workout program. The usual recommendation is to begin with one to two sets of eight to twelve repetitions for each muscle targeted, and do these two to three times a week. Because lifting heavy weights places sudden, intense pressure on your heart and arteries, check with your doctor before doing resistance training to make sure it's okay for you, especially if you have high blood pressure or heart disease.

Cross-training: To prevent boredom, reduce your risk for injury, and ensure that you get the most from your exercise program, try cross-training. Combine two or more types of activity while you

Figure 25: **Bicep Curls**
Stand or sit comfortably with your arms at your sides. Hold a dumbbell in each hand. Bending your elbows, slowly lift the weights to the level of your upper chest, keeping your arms close to your sides. Lower the weights slowly. Repeat. Alternate the position of your hands, first facing your palms forward, then backward (reverse curl).

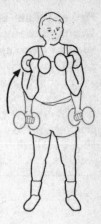

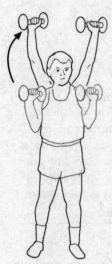

Figure 26: **Military Press**
Stand with your feet slightly apart. Hold a dumbbell in each hand at shoulder height. With your palms facing away from your body, slowly lift the weight upward until your arms are fully extended, then slowly lower the dumbbells to chest level.

Figure 27: **Upright Row**
Stand with your feet at shoulder width. Hold a dumbbell in each hand with your palms facing your thighs. Slowly lift the dumbbells to shoulder level, keeping them close together by allowing your elbows to point outward. Slowly lower the dumbbells to your thighs.

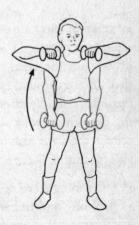

Figure 28: **Knee Extension**
Wearing ankle weights, sit with your knees six inches apart. Place a small rolled towel below the thigh of the leg you will work first. Slowly raise that foot, extending your leg until your knee is as straight as possible. Flex your foot, pointing your toes back toward you. Pause. Relax the foot. Lower it to the floor.

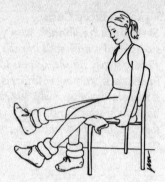

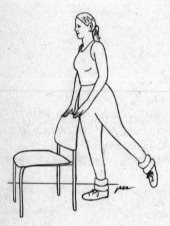

Figure 29: **Hip Extension**
Wearing ankle weights, hold on to a chair back and slowly raise one leg straight out behind you. Lift the leg as high as possible without bending your knee or lowering your upper body forward more than 45 degrees. Pause. Slowly lower your leg.

exercise, or alternate exercises on different days. You can combine stretching with brisk walking, or take a bicycle ride one day and lift weights the next. Mixing activities up in this way will ensure that different muscles are being exercised as you improve your flexibility, muscle strength, and cardiovascular capacity. By varying the parts of your body you exercise at different times, you also reduce the wear and tear on any one area, thereby reducing the risk for injury. Some simple ways to cross-train include:

- Swimming (aerobic exercise) followed by stretching (flexibility)
- Bicycling and treadmill walking in the same session (aerobic) followed by sit-ups (muscle strengthening)

TABLE 21

YOUR EXERCISE PRESCRIPTION

Exercise Type	Duration	Frequency
Warm-up	5–10 minutes	Whenever you exercise
Aerobics	20–60 minutes	3–5 times/week
Muscle toning	15–30 minutes; 1–2 sets of 8–12 repetitions	2–3 times/week
Cooldown	5–10 minutes	Whenever you exercise

Take it slow and build toward these goals gradually. As you incorporate exercise into your life it won't seem so overwhelming—and you'll actually look forward to it.

- Yoga (flexibility) after a brisk walk (aerobic)
- Brisk walk one day (aerobic), weight lifting the next (muscle strengthening)

■ Gauge Your Intensity

The greatest health benefits are gained from exercise done at moderate intensity. There are two ways to gauge your exercise intensity: by heart rate and perceived exertion.

Heart rate: You can measure your heart rate by taking your pulse at your wrist or neck. Before exercising, sit quietly and count the heartbeats (the pulses) for fifteen seconds. Then multiply that number by four to get beats per minute. This gives you your resting heart rate (RHR). To find your exercise heart rate (EHR), exercise until you reach your regular moderate intensity and measure your pulse again. (If you can't take your pulse while moving, stop and check your pulse immediately.) Again, count heartbeats for fifteen seconds and multiply by four.

SIDEBAR 42

HEART-HEALTHY TIP

Aim to accumulate a minimum of three to four hours of exercise and physical activity a week. So if you are doing three 30-minute walks and two 20-minute resistance training workouts a week, that's great, but that only adds up to a little more than two hours. You'll still need to add fifty to sixty minutes of activity (which can be in the form of gardening, mowing the lawn, and so on).

Moderate to vigorous activity increases heart rate to 50 to 85 percent of maximum heart rate (MHR), the heart rate you attain when exercising as hard as you can. For most people, aiming to increase heart rate to 50 to 75 percent of MHR is a reasonable goal; even increasing your heart rate to 40 percent of MHR will provide some benefits. The Karvonen formula is a good way to calculate your target EHR range. (See Table 22, page 235, for details.) However, if you take heart medications such as beta-blockers or calcium channel blockers, this formula will not be accurate for you. Instead, your physician or cardiac-wellness provider can calculate your EHR range based on your performance during a supervised exercise test, usually on a treadmill. An EHR calculated in this way is valid as long as you follow your normal medication regimen. Once you know your EHR range, then you can check your heart rate while you are exercising to determine if you are staying within the recommended range.

In addition to checking for your EHR, you have another option for determining intensity: perceived exertion.

Perceived exertion: Another way to gauge the intensity of your exercise is through perceived exertion. Rather than doing a mathematical calculation, pay attention to how you feel. Signs and symp-

---

TABLE 22

Karvonen Formula

$[(220 - \text{age})* - \text{RHR}] \times \%$ exercise intensity $+ \text{RHR} = \text{EHR}$

Say you are 40 years old and your RHR is 80, and you are aiming for a 50 to 75 percent exercise intensity. Fill in the numbers using the formula above, calculating it in stages:

Step 1: [(220 − age) − RHR]
$[(220 - 40) - 80] = 100$

Step 2: [100] × % (where the % you are aiming for is 50 to 75)
$100 \times 50\% = 50 \qquad 100 \times 75\% = 75$

Step 3: Add RHR
$50 + 80 = 130; 75 + 80 = 155$

Your target EHR is between 130 and 155 beats per minute.

---

*The Karvonen formula uses maximum heart rate (MHR), but the formula we've provided (220 − age) represents a close estimate of MHR for most people.

---

toms to watch for include aches, cramps, pain, fatigue, breathing rate, and shortness of breath. An easy rule of thumb is the "talk test." You should be able to talk and exercise at the same time. If you have trouble talking, you are probably working too hard. However, if you can sing, then you are not working hard enough! (Some exercise programs may suggest interval training with short bursts of extreme intensity during which you can't talk comfortably, but we don't recommend this for most cardiac patients.) Some shortness of breath is natural; you are challenging your body and asking it to get more oxygen into your system more quickly.

You should also feel comfortably fatigued. You should feel challenged, but not overwhelmed. You should feel tired, but not as if you need to stop in another minute or so. And when you finish exercising, you should feel as if you probably could have done more if necessary.

This method is particularly useful in mind/body exercise because it helps you to become more attuned to your body's response to exertion; studies show that how you feel directly relates to your heart rate. With increased body awareness, you can adjust your exercise practice on a day-to-day basis, making the activity more enjoyable, decreasing the risk for injury, and increasing the likelihood that you will continue to do the activity.

The ideal approach, of course, is to use both your heart rate and perceived exertion to determine how much you should exercise at any given time. This is important not only with formal exercise but also with activities related to daily living. Be aware of your exertion level to help pace your activities, to know when to rest or

TABLE 23

PERCEIVED EXERTION

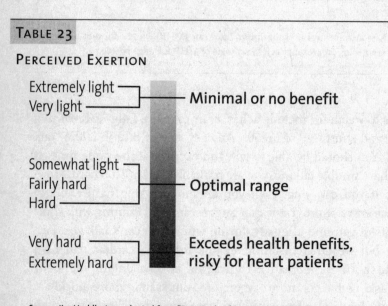

Extremely light / Very light	Minimal or no benefit
Somewhat light / Fairly hard / Hard	Optimal range
Very hard / Extremely hard	Exceeds health benefits, risky for heart patients

Source: Jim Huddleston, adapted from "Borg Scale of Perceived Exertion," from G. A. Borg: "Psychophysical Basis of Perceived Exertion," Medicine and Science in Sports and Exercise 14 (1982): 377.

SIDEBAR 43

EXERCISE SAFETY TIPS

- Drink water! Your body needs to replenish fluids lost during exercise. Drink a glass of water fifteen to thirty minutes before you exercise. On particularly hot days, take a drink every fifteen to twenty minutes while exercising.
- Wear proper shoes. A good supportive shoe is fine for general physical activity, but as you increase the intensity of your exercise, you may need to get more appropriate footwear. Many stores offer shoes and sneakers designed specially for various activities such as walking, jogging, and tennis. They're worth the investment.
- Dress smart. If exercising indoors or in a warm environment, choose lightweight, blended fabrics that will help to wick away moisture. Cotton fabrics are not the best choice since they absorb moisture and retain it, so that you'll feel sticky and sweaty. In cold weather, wear several layers of light clothing: an inner layer of lightweight synthetic fabric to wick away moisture; a middle layer to provide insulation, if necessary; and an outer layer that fits loosely and offers protection against the elements.

ask for help when lifting and moving objects. Depending on the severity of your heart disease, some activities (such as shoveling, lifting heavy objects, and mowing the lawn) may be too strenuous. Talk with your doctor or health care team for guidance about daily activities you can perform safely. Remember, the objective is to feel better, not worse.

■ Remember to Warm Up and Cool Down

Take five to ten minutes both before and after engaging in any moderate to vigorous activity to warm up and cool down. This allows you to loosen and stretch muscles that may feel tight. A warm-up and cool-down routine reduces muscle soreness, allows your heart and blood vessels to adjust to (or recover from) the increased demands of exercise, and reduces the chance of injury during and after exercise or muscle soreness afterward.

Warm up: This will help you prepare for the transition from rest to exercise by increasing blood flow, respiration, and body temperature, and by stretching muscles. To warm up, do a series of gentle stretches, focusing on one muscle group at a time. Hold the position for at least fifteen to twenty seconds to stretch the muscle. Another good way to warm up is to do your preferred aerobic activity at a slow pace so that you ease into it. If you want to take a brisk walk, for instance, spend five minutes walking at a slow speed to let your body progress at its own pace. As you go through a warm-up routine, your body should literally feel warmer as well as more nimble and flexible.

Cool down: Just as important as warming up, spend five to ten minutes cooling down after you complete your exercise. Although this involves much the same process as a warm-up routine, the objective now is to let your body cool off gradually by reducing the intensity of your movements. The cool-down period is especially important for people with heart disease. Stretching and slow movement help to:

- Increase the elasticity of your muscles
- Prevent blood from pooling in any part of your body
- Allow for a gradual dissipation of the body heat and lactic acid that builds up in working muscles and can cause muscle soreness
- Reduce the chance of having irregular heartbeats

As a result of cooling down, you are less likely to feel lightheaded, fatigued, or sore, and you are less likely to injure yourself.

The cool-down period is also a good time to combine movement with relaxation skills.

Elicit the relaxation response: Both warm-up and cool-down routines provide an opportunity to become more mindful of your body, as well as to transition into and out of a more physically active state. As we discussed in Chapter 3, yoga is an excellent way to stretch mindfully and to elicit the relaxation response. The sun salute is especially useful in this regard. We recommend that patients who are able to do the sun salute use it to warm up and cool down because it:

- Puts both your spinal cord and rib cage through a full range of motion, thereby improving flexibility and breathing capacity
- Improves muscle strength, flexibility, and endurance
- Enhances circulation and increases your energy and vitality

At the same time, these rhythmic, gentle motions help quiet the mind. (See pages 79 to 80 for instructions on how to perform the sun salute.)

■ Lose Weight the Mind/Body Way

If you are interested in losing weight, the bottom line is that you must burn more calories in the course of a day than you consume. "Miracle" diets that promise you will shed pounds without a drop of sweat are more hype than help. The only way to lose weight and keep it off is to make a long-term commitment to a new way of eating and exercising; you need to reduce your total calorie count (as we discussed in Chapter 7) while increasing your activity level.

Fortunately, you can lose weight by building on the foundation of fitness we've already described. Continue to exercise at moderate intensity, but increase the frequency and duration of your activities. Also look for ways to include extra bouts of physical ac-

---

SIDEBAR 44

PRESCRIPTION FOR WEIGHT LOSS

To maximize your chances of losing weight, aim for the following:

- Exercise for forty to sixty minutes a day (enough to burn 300–400 calories a session).
- Choose moderate-intensity activities.
- Exercise four to seven times a week (the higher the frequency, the more important that you cross-train to decrease your risk for injury).
- Pick activities that involve large muscle groups such as legs, rather than smaller muscles such as arms.
- Include weight training as well as aerobic activities.

---

tivity in your day in addition to the time you formally set aside for exercise. Like pennies saved, all that physical activity builds up more than you'd think.

■ Change Your Relationship with Exercise

Although losing weight may seem too difficult it is possible. We discussed a mind/body approach to eating better in Chapter 7. You can also apply a mind/body strategy to increasing your physical activity. All this requires is a few adjustments in your attitude.

Love it and lose it: Because losing weight involves exercising on a regular basis for extended periods of time, it is very important that you enjoy whatever activity you choose. Think carefully about what types of physical activities you like to do, and then figure out how to do them more often or at a greater intensity. If you like to walk, for instance, continue to do so—but pick up the pace and gradually add minutes. Don't go to the gym if you feel intimidated by gyms, because chances are at some point you'll get discouraged and stop going.

Learn as you burn: Few people realize how much learning potential there is in physical activity; the benefits go well beyond physical fitness. As you embrace a lifestyle that involves more physical activity and mindfulness, you will stop concentrating on the mechanics of exercise and more on what it means to move. You can spend time meditating and "going with the flow" of your thoughts. What you learn may surprise you. You may gain an appreciation of how your body feels as it moves. Or you may come up with a creative solution to a challenge you've been mulling over. If you are active outdoors, you may notice beauty in nature for the first time. You may also discover how your mind quiets and negative thoughts fade as you focus on your body.

Moderation is best: Although many people think the way to lose weight is to immediately ratchet up the intensity level, studies suggest otherwise. Moderate activities are actually best because you will more likely continue doing them over an extended period of time. (People who exercise so hard that they become exhausted tend to burn out, stop exercising, and gain any lost pounds back again.) So pick moderate-intensity activities, and just try to do them a little longer each day.

Lose weight by lifting weights: Although aerobic exercise is the type that uses fat stores as an energy source and then depletes them, you should also include muscle toning and resistance exercises to your weekly routine. Weight training builds muscle tissue, which is metabolically more active than fat. As a result, muscle not only requires more calories to function but also helps you to burn more calories throughout the day.

■ Special Advice for Women

If you are a woman, you may have to work a little harder at weight loss than a man does, for both physiologic and metabolic reasons. Although women do tend to add more body fat than men over the years (for reasons we'll outline below), research shows that this is due more to a decline in physical activity and overall aerobic capacity than to any underlying difference between the sexes. Women and men who remain physically active are able to significantly reduce the amount of body fat and inches gained as they age.

Fat storage and metabolism: Women tend to store fat in their hips, thighs, and buttocks. This is the hardest type of fat to lose, since fat metabolism in this part of the body is less robust than in the upper abdominal region (where men tend to store fat). It is possible for women to lose fat, but it will take more effort.

Resting metabolism is lower: Women tend to have a resting metabolic rate that is 5 to 10 percent lower than that in men. Resting metabolism helps to determine how quickly you burn calories. Because of their lower metabolic rate, women tend to burn calories more slowly.

Higher percentage of body fat: Women also have a higher percentage of body fat—and lower percentage of lean body mass—compared to men of similar weight. The average American woman has 36 percent body fat, while the typical man has 23 percent. (The amounts considered normal are about half those: 18 to 22 percent for women and 12 to 15 percent for men.) Since muscle burns more calories than fat, this type of body composition also slows weight loss in women.

Caloric expenditure with exercise: Due to their lower resting metabolism and higher percentage of body fat, women, when they exercise, burn up to 40 percent fewer calories than men who do the same activity. Women therefore may have to exercise for a longer period of time to facilitate weight loss.

■ Special Tips for People with Diabetes

If you have diabetes, regular exercise should be as much a part of your treatment as diet and medication. Although you face specific risks, there are ways to minimize them so that you still benefit from exercise.

Blood sugar problems: People with insulin dependent diabetes especially must use caution when exercising, because the injected form of insulin does not decrease naturally as physical activity increases in the way that the natural hormone does. As a result, people who inject insulin may develop low blood sugar during physical activity. Monitor your blood sugar closely and adjust your intake of carbohydrates (and/or your dose of injected insulin) both before and after exercise to prevent low or abnormally high blood sugar levels. You should not exercise if your blood sugar levels are consistently elevated. People who have the more common form of the disease, non-insulin dependent diabetes, also need to pay attention to their blood sugar as they exercise, particularly if they take an oral hypoglycemic medication. Such a medication may facilitate the uptake of glucose into cells, which could lower blood glucose during exercise.

Vascular problems: Vascular changes caused by diabetes can also cause problems during exertion, so avoid particular activities. Fragile eye vessels could rupture, for instance (a problem known as retinopathy), especially if exertion causes a disproportionate rise in blood pressure. People who have peripheral neuropathy—a nerve dysfunction causing pain, numbness, or tingling in the extremities—may injure themselves while exercising without realizing it due to a loss of sensation. It's best to avoid high-impact activities, such as running or basketball, which can injure the feet or hands.

We recommend the following precautions to our patients who have diabetes:

- Consult with your physician, ophthalmologist, and podiatrist before beginning an exercise regimen.
- Monitor your blood sugar level both before and twenty to thirty minutes after exercise to determine how exercise has affected it.
- Avoid doing exercise if your blood sugar level is higher than 250 mg/dL and your urine tests positive for other biological markers known as ketones. Use caution if your blood sugar level is higher than 300 mg/dL and your urine tests negative for ketones. Ketosis results when there is not enough insulin to allow glucose to be used for energy, and the body has to rely exclusively on fat for energy needs. Ketosis is more likely to occur in people with insulin-dependent diabetes.
- Be familiar with the general management of diabetes and the interaction of diet, exercise, and insulin.
- If possible, exercise not too long after having a meal or snack, since having carbohydrates in your system will help stabilize blood sugar levels during exercise.
- Know when your insulin dose hits its peak, and avoid exercising at that time.
- Consider reducing your insulin dose before exercising, depending on the type of insulin and time of day you exercise.
- Watch out for a hypoglycemic "lag effect" that can occur twenty-four to forty-eight hours after exercise; an extra snack after exercise will help.
- Avoid injecting insulin into a muscle that will be active while you exercise.
- Use proper footwear and inspect your feet often to avoid blisters or sores that will be slow to heal.

- Avoid high-impact activities if you are prone to neuropathy in your legs or feet, or if you have a history of retinopathy.
- If you have a history of eye or kidney disease, avoid strenuous weight training and any exercise that involves straining, jarring, or forced breath-holding, as these may increase blood pressure significantly.
- Practice aerobic exercise that emphasizes frequency and duration but is moderate in intensity.
- Avoid high-intensity anaerobic exercise, such as strenuous calisthenics or weight lifting.
- Wear some form of diabetes identification in case you need medical attention.
- Carry a concentrated form of carbohydrates (sugar packets, glucose tablets, or candy such as Life Savers) when exercising, in the event of low blood sugar.

■ Getting Started

Now that we've explained the many benefits of exercise and ways that you can enhance your own fitness level, it's time to get started. Here are some tips on how to do so.

Identify your motive: What is your main reason for wanting to develop a more active lifestyle? The answer is different for everyone. Spend some quiet time thinking about why you personally want to become more physically fit. Some typical reasons include:

- Activity will help me feel better.
- I want to lose weight.
- I want to look better.
- I don't want to have a heart attack.
- I want to be able to play with my grandchildren.
- I enjoy working out with people at an exercise club.
- I enjoy the time I give myself and enjoy getting to know myself better.

There are as many motivations for getting into shape as there are people. Most important is to focus on the reason that is most powerful for you. This is your core motivation. If you find that you are getting discouraged or stop exercising altogether, remind yourself of your core desire. This is usually enough to help get you back on track.

Overcome internal barriers: Ask people about exercise, and often what you get are complaints. Some people find health clubs intimidating and don't want to go near them. Some remember unpleasant childhood experiences involving team sports or exercise. Some people don't want to sweat, especially older women who find it unfeminine. Others yet are overwhelmed at the thought of starting to exercise after a lifetime of being sedentary. The biggest complaint, though, is lack of time. If so, consider this:

According to nineteenth-century English statesman Edward Stanley, "Those who think they have not time for bodily exercise will sooner or later have to find time for illness."

Internal barriers exist because we allow them to remain. Challenge your assumptions. Lack of time, for instance, should not be an excuse. In a twenty-four-hour day, surely there are thirty minutes you can spend on physical activity—especially when you can break that activity down into three ten-minute segments.

Second, if you have a knee-jerk reaction against exercise, think about why you do. Is your own cognitive distortion preventing you from being open to a new type of exercise? (For more on cognitive distortions, see Chapter 4.) Remember that jumping to conclusions is not a form of exercise!

Set reasonable goals: Behavior change takes time, so start slowly and build gradually. Do not attempt any physical activity that feels more demanding than what you can handle. Set reasonable goals and stick to the plan.

Find joy in the process: Although goals are important, so is enjoying yourself. Focus more on the process of an activity, rather than on the outcome. Once you have set your goals, don't fixate on them; instead focus on the experiences you have while getting there. As the philosopher Alan Watts once said, "You don't dance to get to the other side of the floor."

Respect the experience of comfort: Allow activity to happen. Don't force it. Pay attention to your heart rate and your perceived body sensations. Moderation is key. Focus on your breath rhythm and your form. (For safety tips, especially if you have heart disease, see Sidebar 41, page 225.)

Assert your individuality: Whatever you do, remember that you are a unique individual with particular interests, limitations, and challenges. You are the one who is going to do the exercise, so you should find an activity you enjoy and a plan that you can fit comfortably into your life.

Develop a positive attitude: Challenge your old beliefs and turn declarative statements on their head. For example, instead of saying that exercise makes you tired, say that it gives you more energy so that you can get things done with less effort and have more time to spare for leisure and hobbies.

Deal with the details: Plan what you want to do, where, and with whom. Consider any costs involved and what equipment and clothing you need. Planning helps to ensure that you will be ready to start.

Be flexible: Avoid all-or-nothing thinking. Instead, go with the flow. On some days you may want to be more active than on others. Listen to your body, and if you feel tired, then take it easy.

Write a contract: Some people find it helpful to put their intentions and exercise goals in writing. If you find this helps, write down your motivations and goals, and reread your contract when you find your spirit flagging.

It's okay to be happy: Sometimes people who have low self-esteem don't feel worthy of doing something good for themselves. It's as if they don't think they are good enough to feel healthy and happy. This may get in the way of developing heart-healthy habits such as exercising. One way to counter low self-esteem is to think about yourself more positively and make positive statements.

SIDEBAR 45

MARY'S STORY

Mary entered our Cardiac Wellness Program in her early forties, suffering from high blood pressure and occasional incidents of angina. She was obese, weighing almost 250 pounds, with a dangerous BMI of 43. Although Mary took medication to control her blood pressure, she knew she had to lose weight and adopt healthy behaviors if she wanted to see her two young children grow up. But when it came to exercise, she was skeptical.

"I hate exercise," she told us bluntly. "Even as a child I hated exercise. Besides, I don't like to sweat." Mary also felt she was already too squeezed for time. She juggled a demanding job as a teacher with child care arrangements and regular visits to her aging parents. "Why even try to exercise if you can't do thirty minutes in a row?" she asked.

Mary had cultivated some of the most common barriers to exercise. She still associated physical activity with bad childhood memories of being picked last for sports teams. Like some women—and men—Mary did not like the physical sensation of sweating. And like many people, Mary felt like she had no time to exercise.

We advised Mary to start slowly—a fifteen-minute walk, five times a week—and to just try to enjoy herself and keep the pace comfortable. When she felt ready to gradually increase her walking pace and time, she should do so until she was walking at a brisk pace for forty to sixty minutes, three to five times a week (at which point she'd be getting the recommended three to four hours of moderate physical activity a week).

Mary struggled at first. She walked three days one week, for twenty minutes at a time, but then got discouraged and stopped. We asked that Mary challenge some of her cognitive distortions about exercise, especially her all-or-nothing view that it was thirty minutes a day or no walking at all. Mary reframed the issue ("something is better than nothing") and took it more slowly, starting with ten-minute walks. We also suggested that she use her walks as a time to elicit the relaxation response so that she could combine exercise with quiet time.

It took a while, but Mary gradually began to walk regularly and for progressively longer amounts of time. After a month, she was walking four times a week for fifteen to twenty minutes at a time. By the end of the second month, she was walking at least five days a week for thirty minutes at a time (and sometimes longer). To her surprise, she had begun to look forward to these walks and even said she enjoyed them. By the third month, just before she finished the Cardiac Wellness Program, Mary was walking five to seven times a week for forty-five to sixty minutes at a time. She now enjoyed it so much that she had joined the Appalachian Mountain Club, which sponsors outdoor walks and hikes for people along the East Coast. Mary felt she had developed a new relationship with exercise.

■ Keep Going

It is the rare person who becomes more physically active without a hitch. Most people get discouraged and find their spirits flagging, especially in the beginning. If this happens to you, consider the following strategies.

Rethink success: Often we approach exercise with the kind of all-or-nothing thinking discussed in Chapter 4 along with other examples of cognitive distortions. According to this line of thinking, if we stop exercising for one or two days, then we have failed.

It's time to rethink your definition of success. People who are trying for the first time to integrate physical activity into their life often progress in a cyclical way, rather than in a linear progression. It's normal to make progress, then get off track for a while, then start exercising again. Every step you take is a step in the right direction. Support helps. Seek company: You don't have to "go it alone." Walking with a friend can provide the encouragement you need at the beginning.

Listen to your body: To get started, you may have to say to yourself, "Just do it." Once you have started, however, remember to listen to your body. This will help you make better choices while exercising, decrease your risk for injury, and improve your chances of long-term success. The intensity of your exercise or the length of time you spend may vary from day to day—just as your moods, needs, and energy levels do. Your mental focus may also vary. Some days you may want to focus on the more physical aspects of the exercise, pushing yourself harder. Other days you may want to quiet your mind and relax or let your thoughts flow freely if you are in a creative mood. Listen to your innermost self as well as to the signals you receive from your body (relating to energy, fatigue, tension release). By listening to your body and heeding the messages it sends, you can adjust your exercise practice to enhance your psychological, emotional, and physical health.

Keep up the momentum: Family vacations and visitors can sometimes interrupt your exercise routine, and it may be hard to get started again afterward. Before a holiday, consider alternatives to your usual routine. Be creative. Let's say you've been working out at a local health club but plan to go away camping for two weeks. Can you walk, hike, or swim at the campsite? If friends are visiting from out of town, invite them to exercise with you—or let them know you'll need time each day to do it yourself.

Variety is the spice of life: Vary your exercise routine through cross-training. (See page 230.) This helps prevent boredom, decreases the chances that you will injure yourself, results in overall better conditioning, and increases the "fun factor." Think of different activities you can do throughout the week. Increasing variety will help motivate you to continue and will prevent barriers from getting in the way.

No one is perfect: Aim for a lifetime of physical activity, but remember that no one is perfect. If you find yourself slipping from your exercise habit, instead of beating yourself up, look at it as a learning experience. What happened? Why did you stop exercising? What got in the way? Can you prevent it from happening again? The answers to these questions will help you get back on track and stay there.

Keep plugging: Remember that any behavior change takes time. Give yourself at least six months, and expect some ups and downs as you progress in the cyclical fashion we discussed earlier. If you slip a bit, get going again. If you keep at it, at some point you will wake up and realize that you want to exercise. At that point, exercise will have become an integral part of your life.

Reward yourself: Adults are not that much different from children. We all like to be recognized for a job well done. So if you have met one of your goals for exercise, acknowledge that achievement. Celebrate! And then keep moving.

■ Putting It All Together

As you consider different ways to become physically active, we'd like to suggest two activities that are a great way to get started and will help to pull the various threads of this chapter together. Both can also be used to elicit the relaxation response, which is the foundation of our Cardiac Wellness Program.

■ Tai Chi Sample Practice

Although Tai Chi originated as a form of martial arts and self-defense, it has evolved into a practice that emphasizes unity of mind, body, and spirit, while fostering a harmonious connection to the environment. The gentle, slow, almost dancelike movements encourage an inner stillness and focus on the present moment that is helpful in eliciting the relaxation response. Yet this ancient Chinese practice also involves a moderate-intensity exercise that:

- Improves cardiovascular health
- Bolsters immune system function
- Increases flexibility and muscle strength
- Improves coordination and balance, thereby reducing risk for falls and injury

The following sequence can help you experience the spiritual and physical benefits of Tai Chi, as you visualize your energy (qi) aligned with the fundamental elements of life: wood, fire, earth, metal, and water.

1. To begin, stand comfortably, take a few deep breaths, and relax, focusing on the rhythm of your breathing.
2. Let your legs relax so that you sink slightly downward, toward the earth, to connect with the energy of your environment.

3. Raise your arms out to the side, about shoulder level, as if opening yourself up to the universe.

4. Form a circle with your arms by touching your fingers in front of you, as if you were embracing the earth and bringing energy to your heart.

5. Take a step backward while opening your arms, as if you were a flower blooming or a tree sprouting branches. Move your arms gently, as if a breeze were blowing your arms in the wind.

6. Come to center with your hands, then stretch one arm up toward the sky and the other down toward the earth. Repeat, switching arms as you do, and gently increase the length of the stretch. (If you feel like you need to stretch more, repeat several times.)

7. Make circles with your arms, while bringing them slowly back to the center of your body, making progressively smaller circles as you go and ending at your navel. With one hand resting on top of another, make small circular motions with your hands, as if rubbing your stomach. (The circles stimulate the circulation of energy; according to Taoist precepts, we are born from the navel and our life energy, or *qi*, resides there.)

8. Pull your forward leg back, and step forward, reaching both arms forward and up to the sky. You are simulating fire now, releasing a powerful burst of energy.

9. Slowly bring your arms back down to shoulder level, mimicking rain falling from the sky. As your hands move back toward the earth, imagine the cooling water nourishing the roots of a tree so that it will grow strong.

10. Begin to turn slowly in half circles, as if you were a tree gently swaying in the wind. Reverse direction and turn in a full circle; as you turn, notice the elements of nature around you: the sun, trees, vegetation, the feel of the air on your skin.

11. As you face forward, swing one arm up and back to front (a bit like doing backstroke), as if you were trying to capture the world's energy.

12. As your arm swings to the front, continue the arc and imagine that you are reaching for a crystal above your head and then moving it downward, drawing energy from your head to your heart to your navel, pulling all that energy toward you. Say *"ching"* softly as you do so, to help clear and purify the central channel through which your *qi* flows. Repeat with your other arm.

13. Bend both knees and let both arms drop to the ground, as you visualize letting go of burdens in your life. (You can even softly say *"let go."*)

14. Raise your arms toward the sun, feeling much lighter now. Absorb the energy of the sun.

15. Position your palms downward and slowly lower your arms at your sides, squatting slightly, as you reconnect with the earth's energy.

16. Bring your arms together in front of you and slowly raise them to neck level, as if you were scooping up the earth's energy and drawing it through your entire body.

17. Continue to move your arms so that you stretch them upward to the sky, as if you were exploding with all this good energy. Introduce yourself to the world: "Here I am, as I am."

18. Gently lower your arms and cross your hands at heart level so that you create a small private space between your hands and your heart. Focus on this space. You have now brought a balance of yin (the female elements) and yang (male)—and of things you desire and do not desire—to your heart.

19. Stand with your feet comfortably apart and push your hands down toward the earth, squatting slightly, returning energy to the ground beneath you.

19. Stand up straight, rising from the earth, to end the sequence.

■ Mindful Walking

Another good activity is mindful walking, which combines the Western need to do something (walk) and the Eastern need simply to be (pray, meditate). Mindful walking satisfies the body's need to exercise and the soul's need to relax and reflect. It represents the coexistence of inner silence and outer activity. As such, mindful walking is exercise for the whole person. Similar in philosophy to yoga, mindful walking involves every part of us: mind, body, and spirit (or soul). It integrates parts of ourselves that may ordinarily be fragmented.

The key to mindful walking is mindfulness: the ability to focus on only the thing you are currently doing (in this case, walking). As the Buddhist philosopher Thich Nhat Hanh once wrote, "Mindfulness is the miracle by which we call back in a flash our dispersed mind and restore it to wholeness so that we can live each moment of life."

Mindful walking is not just about getting to a destination. It is about process rather than outcome. "To travel hopefully is a better thing than to arrive," as the poet Robert Louis Stevenson put it.

■ Suggestions for Mindful Walking

The best approach to mindful walking is the one that works for you. Be flexible and open to all possibilities. No matter what technique you use, your attention will likely drift at times. Just acknowledge the distracting thoughts, much as you would clouds in the sky, let (watch) them go and then refocus. Here are some tips on how to walk mindfully:

- Focus on your breathing. Breathe deeply through your nose. Breathe in the good (energy, awareness, love, peace, serenity) and breathe out the bad (frustrations, distractions, fear, pain).

SAMPLE PRAYERS FOR MINDFUL WALKING

Many religions offer prayers that may help you maintain a spiritual focus as you walk mindfully. Several examples follow:

NAVAJO PRAYER
With beauty before me may I walk,
With beauty behind me may I walk,
With beauty above me may I walk,
With beauty all around me may I walk.

In old age wandering on a trail of beauty,
Lively may I walk;
In old age wandering on a trail of beauty,
Lively again, may I walk.

It is finished in beauty.

PRAYER FROM BLACK ELK, A LAKOTA MEDICINE MAN
Great Spirit, Great Spirit, My Grandfather
All over the earth the faces of living things are all alike.
With tenderness have these come up out of the ground.
Look upon these faces of children without number
And with children in their arms,
That they may face the winds
And walk the good road to the day of quiet.

SCRIPTURAL PASSAGES
Isaiah (2:3–4)
Come, let us go to the mountain of the Lord,
To the house of the God of Jacob;
That he may teach us his ways
And that we may walk in his paths.

Micah (4:5)
For all the people walk,
Each in the name of its god,
But we will walk
In the name of the Lord our God
Forever and ever.

- Pay attention to the cadence of your steps as you walk. Steps can be a physical mantra. Try to coordinate the rhythm of your breathing with the rhythm of your steps. Count to four slowly as you breathe inward, matching each number with a step, and to four again as you exhale.
- Add a mantra or some type of affirmation to your cadence. A three-count cadence (as for a waltz) is slightly less rhythmical than a four-count cadence, and thus may hold your attention more. Some examples of three-count cadences include:

> I am here
> I can walk
> I am strong
> I like me

Or try something more spiritual and nature based:

> Lotus flower blooms.
> The green planet

You can also add spiritual elements, so that your mindful walk becomes a prayer walk. Now you are truly exercising body, mind, and spirit!

Using the tools and advice we have provided in this chapter, develop a rhythm of physical activity that fits into your life. When you make physical activity an integral part of who you are, you have taken a big step toward living a healthier, happier life.

Chapter 9

Making It Work

A tree as great as a man's embrace springs from a small shoot. A terrace nine stories high begins with a pile of earth. A journey of a thousand miles starts under one's feet.

—LAO TZU, CHINESE TAOIST PHILOSOPHER

THROUGHOUT THIS BOOK, we have suggested a number of strategies and techniques that you can use to improve the health of your heart. In this chapter, we'll discuss strategies to help you stay on track in your commitment to your new lifestyle.

Change, after all, is a journey—and it is like any journey, filled with unexpected twists and turns, challenges that might set you back a few steps, moments of frustration as well as elation. It is the rare person who is able to embrace change without a few setbacks. Most of us take a few steps forward, then a few steps back.

Yet too often in the medical model of illness, people and their behaviors are thought of in black-and-white terms. Either you are cured or you are sick; healthy or unhealthy; in remission from an old habit or relapsed. We don't see it that way. Changing behaviors is a complex process. The main thing is to keep heading in the right direction.

■ Where Are You Now?

First take some time to reassess your goals and values. We introduced several "self-assessment" exercises in Chapter 1 that were intended to provide insight into where you are psychologically, physically, and spiritually. Try doing these exercises again to see if anything has changed now that you've learned more about the mind/body connection and strategies for self-care.

Has your self-portrait changed at all? Are you happy with the way you look in the new picture or do you think you still need to work more on self-care? (To see how some of our patients changed, take a look at their "before" portraits in Chapter 1, page 10, and their "after" self-portraits on page 260.

Now determine what is important to you by repeating the balance exercise on page 11. Have your answers changed now that you've done other exercises in the book? Have you rediscovered something you'd forgotten about? Are you doing the things that you identified as important and meaningful more often?

Finally, draw another time pie. (See pages 11–13.) Has the mix of obligations and pleasures changed in your pie? Are you satisfied with the way you spend your days? Are you taking more time for yourself? Have you built in time for the relaxation response and exercise? Remember, there are no right or wrong answers to these questions. We just want to get you thinking.

■ Revisit Your Health Contract

Remind yourself of where you want to go: What are your long-term goals? Start by reviewing the health contract you filled out in the self-assessment exercise in Chapter 1. (See pages 13–15.) Have you achieved any of the goals you identified earlier? Are you making progress? If not, what obstacles have you encountered in making these changes? They can be people, old habits, or challenging situations. List them below:

_____

_____

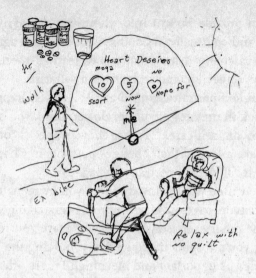

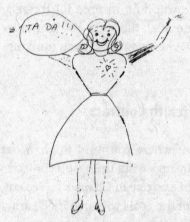

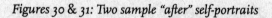

Figures 30 & 31: Two sample "after" self-portraits

Now think about who or what will help you overcome these obstacles. Think about the different types of social support discussed in Chapters 4 and 5. Your support might come from friends, family, coworkers, hobbies, spiritual worship, or physical activity. List your supports below:

_____

_____

Finally, draw up a new health contract. Some goals may remain the same; you may revise others based on your experiences or to vary the routine. Plan to revisit this health contract every six months or so and make revisions as necessary.

▨ Revised Health Contract

GOAL 1: LEARN HOW TO BETTER MANAGE STRESS AND EMOTIONS IN DAILY LIFE.

Read Chapters 3, 4, and 5 to help you with this section.
- Practice the relaxation response.
  Method: _____
  Frequency: _____ Duration: _____
  Find a quiet place where you will not be disturbed.
- Practice three to four "minis" every day.
- Try to spend time each day thinking about the small things in life that can bring you pleasure: watching a sunset, taking a warm bath, enjoying a candlelit dinner or a walk with a friend. Identify some of your own: _____

- Focus on areas in your life that *are* going well as much as you do on those that are not going well.

  Stop: The next time you feel stressed, simply say "stop" to yourself. This stops the negative stress cycle from escalating into a worst-case scenario.

Breathe: Take a couple of slow, deep diaphragmatic breaths. This reduces physical tension and helps you to relax.

Reflect: Notice how you feel (What are your stress warning signs?). Identify your automatic thoughts. Use the cognitive restructuring log (Table 8, pages 110–113). What distortions do your automatic thoughts contain?

Choose: Challenge your automatic way of thinking. How else can I think about this situation and what else can I do to help me cope better? Try to change each automatic thought to a more positive, realistic statement (It's one step at a time, I am doing the best I can, etc.). Notice how you feel now. The more you practice this process, the easier it gets.

GOAL 2: DEVELOP AN EXERCISE PROGRAM THAT IS COMFORTABLE, CHALLENGING, AND ENJOYABLE.

Read Chapter 8 for more information when filling out this section.
Type: _____
Include both aerobic and strength training exercises.
Frequency: _____ Duration: _____
Intensity (measured in heart rate or perceived exertion): _____

- Remember to warm up and cool down for five to ten minutes every time you exercise. These are good times to incorporate the yoga stretches we've included.
- Try to accumulate thirty minutes of brisk physical activity on all or most days of the week. (This includes walking to work and walking for enjoyment, as well as housework, yard work, and regular exercise.)

GOAL 3: DEVELOP A HEART-HEALTHY NUTRITION PLAN.

Read Chapters 2, 6, and 7 for more information.
My starting weight is: _____

My short-term weight goal is: _____
My long-term weight goal is: _____
My latest lipid profile is:
    Date: _____ TC: _____ LDL: _____ HDL: _____ Trigs: _____
    Ideal lipids are TC less than 200, LDL less than 130 (no heart
    disease) or less than 100 (with heart disease or diabetes), HDL
    greater than 40, Trigs less than 150.
My fat-gram goal is 25 to 35 percent of calories a day, and I will
    try to consume more monounsaturated and omega-3 fats
    and less saturated and trans fats.
My sodium goal is a maximum of 2,000 mg a day.
To reach these goals I will:

    1. Balance my plate.
    2. Eat at least five servings of fruits and vegetables a day.
    3. _____
    4. _____
    5. _____

Sample meal plan for the day:

Breakfast
Whole-grain cereal with skim milk and fruit
Coffee or tea

Lunch
Tossed green salad with avocado and several strips of chicken
Oil (unsaturated) and vinegar dressing
Whole wheat roll
Low-calorie beverage

Healthy snack
Cottage by the Cheese (see recipe, page 275)

Dinner
Grilled salmon

Steamed vegetable medley (broccoli, carrots, snow peas,
   tomatoes)
Brown rice
Low-calorie beverage

■ Lapses Are Normal

Recovery is a process, not an event.
—ANNE WILSON SCHAEF, AUTHOR

If you haven't achieved all your goals or have had a few setbacks, don't worry. It's normal to experience occasional lapses as you try to integrate change into your life. A lapse is a single event during which you take up an old behavior you've been trying to change. We've all had them. It's the decision to eat a piece of chocolate cake instead of taking a walk when you've had a hard day. It's reaching for that pack of cigarettes so that you can have "just one." Afterward, you may feel guilty and discouraged. "It's no use; I can't change; I'm a failure" are all common reactions. Yet this all-or-nothing type of thinking is a cognitive distortion and does not mirror reality. (For more on how to overcome cognitive distortions, see Chapter 4.)

The key to overcoming lapses is to expect them on occasion just as traffic tie-ups and road construction may delay you on the highway. Think about the last time you embarked on a long road trip. Chances are, you encountered something along the way that slowed you down—but you did not give up, turn the car around, and head home. You still reached your intended destination, though it may have taken you a little longer than expected.

It's the same with personal change. Let's say you've been trying to become more physically active, but then you go for a whole week without doing any exercise. Or you've been balancing your plate, adding more fruits and vegetables, but suddenly give in to the urge to eat a fast-food hamburger. The world won't end. You've had a lapse—but you're not a failure.

Remind yourself of why you wanted to change in the first place, and then start making progress again and keep at it. Review your values and goals listed in the self-assessment exercises from time to time, just to remind yourself of the direction you'd like to be headed in.

Another good strategy is to identify your negative thinking patterns. Watch for the distortions behind statements like:

I'm a failure.
I can't do this.
I have no willpower.
What's the use?

Reframe your thinking, using the tips that we described in Chapter 4. First, stop, breathe, reflect, and choose. Then try to think differently:

It's just a bump in the road.
I'm doing the best I can.
I can do this.
I am confident.

For more on cognitive restructuring, review stress management advice in Chapter 4.

■ Staying on Track

The real problem for those aiming for change is not the occasional lapse, but a relapse—a complete return to their old heart-risky habits. Although a relapse often seems to happen suddenly, it usually occurs in response to a particular trigger. If you learn how to recognize triggers and plan your response in advance, you will be less likely to relapse.

Drs. Alan Marlatt and Judith R. Gordon, from the University of Washington, found that 75 percent of all relapses stem from one of three scenarios. Although Drs. Marlatt and Gordon identified these situations while researching relapse in addictive behaviors, we think their findings apply to any type of habit that has become ingrained in a person's life.

- Negative emotions, such as anger, boredom, anxiety, frustration, and depression, account for 35 percent of relapses.
- Interpersonal conflicts (with your spouse, friends, boss, or others) cause 20 percent of relapses.
- Social pressure (such as someone who smokes and offers you a cigarette, even though you've quit, or simply observing a particular behavior in others around you) causes about 20 percent of relapses.

■ Tips for Relapse Prevention

Although we can't guarantee that you won't relapse, we can provide strategies that reduce the risk once you've identified the people and situations that may act as triggers.

Avoid triggers: Most negative behaviors are triggered by particular social or physical cues. Avoid these triggers, and you will help to prevent relapse. For instance, if you have quit smoking, avoid bars or other areas where people smoke. Meet friends in the smoke-free section of a restaurant.

Distract yourself: Plan an enjoyable distraction to keep you from reverting to old habits. For instance, if you tend to overeat at night in front of the TV (see page 204, about the overeating chain), try to schedule another activity that will remove the stimulus. Read a book, or meet a friend for an after-dinner walk. Pick something you like to do.

Seek out support: People most likely to maintain change have help: Social support is a vital part of long-term behavior change. Join a support group of people trying to change the same behavior you are.

Think positive: Cheer yourself along with affirmations; negative thinking will only discourage you. Instead of thinking, "I'll never be able to change," say to yourself, "I am stronger than this habit. I can do it."

Resistance through distance: The next time you crave an unhealthy food or have an urge to resume a bad habit, try to observe the urge rather than identifying with it. Instead of saying, "I really want a cigarette," think to yourself, "There's that craving for nicotine again." Creating this type of mental distance helps you to resist the craving until it passes.

Remember the relaxation response: The foundation of our mind/body approach to heart health is the relaxation response. (See Chapter 3.) Remember to build on this foundation. So many relapses are triggered by stress or negative emotions; eliciting the relaxation response on a daily basis can help produce a reservoir of calm that you can draw on throughout the day.

Balance demands with satisfaction: Everyone faces external demands in life. The key to maintaining health is to balance those demands (the things you "should" do) with personal sources of happiness (the things you "want" to do). If you find you are doing all the things you "should" do each day—and not getting to what you want to do—it's time to reevaluate. A good way to reorient yourself is to do a time inventory. (See an example on page 12.)

■ Identify Your Own Strategies

Take time to identify what situations and people will place you at high risk for relapse for a particular behavior. Be specific: Where will this situation take place? Who will be there? And what can you do to avoid a relapse? (Think of a positive response that you will enjoy.)

RELAPSE TRIGGER	WHAT I CAN DO TO COPE
(who, what, when . . .)	*(something you enjoy)*
Candy jar at work	*Pack a low-calorie yogurt snack to feed my sweet tooth.*
_____	_____
_____	_____

■ Practice Optimal Self-Care

As you embark on your journey of change, remember that any time you meet a challenge, you should practice the four-step process we described in Chapter 4: Stop, breathe, reflect, and choose. Use the coping skills we've described in the previous chapters. You may find that what first appeared as a threat is actually an opportunity for growth.

The following suggestions may also be helpful. If you find them so, xerox these pages and put them someplace where you can reread them occasionally.

- Find some time during the day to meditate or listen to a relaxation tape.
- Organize your work; set priorities. Make a list daily, then evaluate your various tasks and divide them into three columns: A (must do), B (can wait), and C (let it go).
- Don't try to be perfect. Don't feel like you have to do everything. It's okay to make a mistake. You're only human.
- Don't try to do two or three or more things at a time.
- Reduce the noise level in your work or home environment, if possible. Instead, listen to soothing music.
- Don't take your job home with you or on breaks. If you can't avoid it, at least limit the time you spend worrying. (Some of our patients find it helpful to designate ten minutes a day for worrying only. Then they let it go.)
- Remember to get enough sleep at night.
- Develop with friends and coworkers your own brand of happy hour, parties, birthday celebrations, and other events that break up routine.
- Look at unavoidable stress as an avenue for growth and change.
- Avoid people who are stress carriers or negaholics.
- Adopt a pet.
- Don't watch the 11 P.M. news.
- Praise yourself regularly; give yourself a pat on the back for something you're proud of.
- Develop a wide variety of resources for gratification in your life, whether it's family, friends, hobbies, interests, special weekends, or vacations. Treat yourself to "new and good things."
- Be assertive. Learn to express your needs and differences, to make requests, and to say "no" constructively.
- Don't overlook emotional resources who are close at hand: spouse, friends, family, and coworkers.
- Don't be afraid to ask questions or to ask for help.
- Allow an extra fifteen minutes to get to work or appointments.

- Check your breathing throughout the day. Practice diaphragmatic breathing when you find yourself shifting into upper chest breathing.
- Remember to do at least three to four "minis" a day. Use dots or some other visual aid to remind yourself.
- Humor is a great coping strategy. Try to find something funny in a situation.
- Take a "mental health" day.
- Practice being patient. Create patience practice periods; for example, when waiting in line. Watch your thoughts; focus on your breathing.
- Understand that we do not all see or do things in the same way.
- Practice mindfulness. Learn to live in the moment. Observe nature. Take a mindful walk. Eat mindfully.
- Become a less aggressive driver.
- Create helping rituals. They make you feel good. Open the door for someone; pick up litter, etc.
- When feeling stress, ask yourself, "Is this really important? Will it really matter a week, month, or year from now?"
- Resist the urge to judge or criticize.
- Become a better listener.
- Breathe before speaking; then you won't interrupt or finish other people's sentences.
- Be flexible with change; things don't always go as planned.
- Say a short prayer or observe a moment of silence before meals.
- Practice an affirmation each day:
  - I am relaxed.
  - One day at a time
  - I am doing the best I can.
  - I am healthy and strong.

We hope that the advice and strategies in this book have helped you make changes that improve the health of your heart. Many of our patients have told us that they have come to view heart disease as an opportunity, because it prompted them to take better care of themselves and to take steps to reconnect with people and activities they value most. So whatever strategies you follow, try to find joy in the process. Both your heart and your spirit will benefit.

Tempting Tempeh Stir-Fry (entrée)

1 to 2 8-ounce packages tempeh, sliced in ¼-inch strips
2½ to 3 tablespoons low-sodium tamari sauce
4 cloves garlic, 3 minced, 1 whole
1½ teaspoons grated fresh ginger
1 bunch scallions, chopped
1 tablespoon olive oil
2 carrots, sliced
2 stalks celery, chopped
1 bunch broccoli, chopped
1 green pepper, chopped or cut into strips
1 red pepper, chopped or cut into strips

Marinate tempeh strips in 1½ to 2 tablespoons tamari sauce. This can be done just before cooking if necessary.

Begin stir-fry by sautéing minced garlic, ginger, and scallions in oil in a wok over medium-low heat. As you add more ingredients to wok slowly increase heat to high.

Add one vegetable at a time and stir-fry each at the bottom of the wok for 30 to 60 seconds, before pushing it off to the side to add another vegetable. Start with the carrots, then cook the celery, and then the broccoli. If the pan becomes dry at any time during cooking process, add a few tablespoons of water.

Place tempeh at bottom of wok and stir-fry until it is slightly browned. When done, push off to the side of the wok.

Add and sauté the green pepper, then the red pepper.

Evenly distribute final tablespoon of tamari over all the food in the wok.

Using a garlic press, crush one clove of garlic over the food.

Cover and let steam for a minute. (If the pan is dry, add ⅛ cup water.)

Serve over brown rice.

Yield: 5 servings
For each serving of Tempting Tempeh Stir-Fry:
Calories: 179; Protein: 12 g; Carbohydrates: 23 g; Fiber: 7.5 g;
Sodium: 365 mg; Total fat: 5.5 g; Saturated fat: 0.7 g; Cholesterol:
0 mg
For every ½ cup of cooked brown rice:
Calories: 110; Protein: 2 g; Carbohydrates: 23 g; Fiber: 1.75 g;
Sodium: 1 mg; Total fat: 0.8 g; Saturated fat: 0.1 g; Cholesterol:
0 mg

Bean Burritos (entrée)

Brands selected for low saturated and trans fat content

1 green pepper, chopped
1 onion, chopped
6 Homestyle Kitchen Tortillas
1 19-ounce can black beans, rinsed
3 ounces Dragone Lite Mozzarella Cheese
½ jar Enrico's Salsa, no salt added

Sauté peppers and onions and then divide equally among each tortilla.

Place 2½ tablespoons or more beans and ½ ounce (2 tablespoons) or more cheese in middle of each tortilla.

Fold in each of the tortilla's four sides to make a rectangular burrito.

Repeat above step for the remaining tortillas.

Place burritos in baking pan. Pour ½ jar of salsa evenly over the 6 burritos.

Bake at 350 degrees F for 20 to 25 minutes or until lightly browned.

Serve with low-calorie vegetables or salad.

Yield: 6 servings
For each serving of Bean Burritos:
Calories: 228; Protein: 12 g; Carbohydrates: 38 g; Fiber: 6.3 g;
Sodium: 625 mg; Total fat: 3 g; Saturated fat: 0.5 g; Cholesterol:
< 5 mg

Cottage by the Cheese (appetizer)

16-ounce package fat-free cottage cheese or Hood Light Cottage
Cheese, no salt added
½ red onion, finely diced
1 carrot, finely diced
1 stalk of celery, finely diced

Mix all the ingredients together and serve with low-fat crackers (Wasa, Kavli, Ak-Mak, Woven Wheats) or whole wheat bread.

Yield: 4 servings
For each serving of cheese on two Hearty Rye Wasa Crackers:
Calories: 185; Protein: 16 g; Carbohydrates: 25 g; Fiber: 5 g;
Sodium: 135 mg; Total fat: 1 g; Saturated fat: 0.5 g; Cholesterol:
5 mg

Black Beauty (bean dip snack or appetizer)

1 15-ounce can black beans, drained and rinsed
2 teaspoons plain nonfat yogurt
½ small green hot chili pepper, seeded and minced
1 clove garlic, crushed

1 teaspoon chili powder
3 whole wheat pita pockets or 6 slices whole wheat bread
tomato, onion, and cucumber, sliced

Place the rinsed black beans in a bowl and mash to a pulp with a fork.

Add the yogurt, chili pepper, garlic, and chili powder, and mix to make a uniform spread.

Serve on whole wheat bread or in a pita pocket. Add sliced tomato, onion, and cucumber.

Yield: 6 servings, ¼ cup each
For each serving of Black Beauty bean dip:
Calories: 168; Protein: 9 g; Carbohydrates: 32 g; Fiber: 7.5 g;
Sodium: 257 mg; Total fat: 1 g; Saturated fat: 0 g; Cholesterol:
0 mg

Muesli (snack)

2 cups rolled oats
2 cups skim milk
2 tablespoons dark seedless raisins
1 apple, cored and chopped
1 banana, sliced
1 orange, peeled and cubed
1 tablespoon sliced almonds
1 cup vanilla-flavored light nonfat yogurt

Mix the rolled oats and skim milk before you prepare the other ingredients. Add the other ingredients and mix well. Eat right away or refrigerate for later. (If you make it ahead of time, omit the banana until you are ready to serve the muesli.)

Yield: 8 servings 1 cup each
For each serving of Muesli:
Calories: 160; Protein: 8 g; Carbohydrates: 28 g; Fiber: 3 g;

*Sodium: 47 mg; Total fat: 2 g; Saturated fat: 0 g; Cholesterol:
0 mg*

Yogurt Pie (dessert)

10 cups plain nonfat yogurt (to make 5 cups yogurt cheese)
5 tablespoons sugar or sugar substitute such as Splenda
1 teaspoon vanilla extract
Assorted fresh fruit (berries, pitted cherries, sliced peaches)

To create yogurt cheese:

Place a coffee filter in a strainer or colander, and set over a large
bowl. If using a colander, you may have to line it with a few filters.

Pour plain nonfat yogurt into the filter.

Cover with plastic wrap.

Refrigerate, covered, for 36 to 48 hours. About half of the original
yogurt will become cheese as the liquid fraction, or whey, drips
down into the bowl. Discard the liquid periodically so that it doesn't
back up into the cheese.

You can serve yogurt cheese on its own, or mix in chopped
scallions, green peppers, and herbs for a spread to put on bagels or
bread. It can also be used in desserts, as we have suggested in the
following recipe.

To make trans fat–free crust (makes 2 pie crusts)

⅔ cup canola oil
⅓ cup water
2 cups white flour
½ teaspoon salt

Microwave oil and water together until almost boiling (must be very
hot—about 2 minutes). You can also heat them on the stove if you
prefer. If you accidentally boil the mixture, let it cool a bit before
proceeding.

Add flour and salt to the oil and water.

Quickly stir mixture into a ball.

Cut ball in halves and place each in a pie plate.

Using a large serving spoon, spread out raw dough until it covers bottom of pie plate.

Repeat process for second half of the dough.

To make yogurt pie:

Place the yogurt cheese in a medium-size bowl with sugar and vanilla.

Beat lightly with a whisk until completely blended.

Turn blended mixture into the prepared crust.

Cover tightly with plastic wrap and chill.

Serve with a topping such as fruit.

Yield: 8 servings
For a serving of filling:
Calories: 182; Protein: 14 g; Carbohydrates: 30 g; Fiber: 2 g;
Sodium: 190 mg; Total fat: 0.6 g; Saturated fat: 0.3 g; Cholesterol:
5 mg (Note: These numbers reflect sugar as the sweetener and
2 cups of fresh raspberries on top of the pie. If you use a sugar
substitute you will save 25 calories and 7 g of carbohydrates per
slice.)
For a serving of pie crust:
Calories: 137; Protein: 1.6 g; Carbohydrates: 12 g; Fiber 0.5 g;
Sodium: 73 mg; Total fat: 9 g; Saturated fat: 0.7 mg; Cholesterol:
0 mg

Smoothie (soy milk shake)

1 cup orange juice
1 cup skim or fortified soy milk
3 tablespoons wheat germ

1 cup fresh or frozen fruit (strawberries, blueberries, bananas,
    peaches, etc.)
Pinch of cinnamon

Place all ingredients in blender and puree on high speed until
smooth. Serve immediately or refrigerate to drink later (up to six to
eight hours). If you prepare the shake ahead of time, blend it again
before serving.

Yield: 2 servings, 1¼ cup each
    For each Smoothie:
    Calories: 160; Protein: 8.5 g; Carbohydrates: 20 g; Fiber: 3 g;
    Sodium: 65 mg; Total fat: 1.8 g; Saturated fat: 0 g; Cholesterol:
    2 mg

There are thousands of foods on the shelves of your supermarket. We recommend the following list because these products are more healthful than many of their alternatives:

BEVERAGES
Bottled Water
Canada Dry flavored seltzer water
Poland Springs flavored seltzer water
Polar flavored seltzer water
Juices
Fruit juices (Look for 100 percent fruit juice, Juicy Juice, or
    other brands)
Light 'n Tangy V8
Low-sodium V8 drinks
Other
Fruit$_2$O
Gatorade Propel drinks
Simply Smart milk (creamier than other low-fat milk)
Tea (black, herbal, or green; caffeinated or decaffeinated)
Waist Watchers diet sodas

BREADS, MUFFINS, TORTILLAS, ETC.
Bagels
Trader Joe's Whole Wheat Bagels (Bagel Spinoza)
Bread
Whole-grain breads (any brand; first ingredient should be
    whole wheat flour or whole-grain flour)
The following breads have 2 grams of fiber per slice but only
60–70 calories:

Arnold's Stoneground 100% Whole Wheat Bread
Country Kitchen Stoneground 100% Whole Wheat
   Bread
Matthew's All Natural Whole Wheat Bread
Trader Joe's Sunflower Sesame Seed Bread (whole grain)
Vermont Bread Company whole wheat breads
The following breads are high in fiber (2.5 grams/slice) and
only 40 calories per slice:
Arnold's Bakery Light Italian Bread
Beefsteak Light Soft Rye
Wonder Light Wheat

Muffins and Baked Loaves

Duncan Hines Muffin Mix
English muffins (any brand; oat bran or whole wheat
   preferred)
Gold Medal Golden Corn Muffin Mix (less trans fat compared
   to most but not to whole grain)
Mrs. Crutchfield's Fat-Free Corn Muffins
Pillsbury Quick Bread Mix Cranberry Bread
Trader Joe's Toasted Corn Mini Loaf

Pita Bread

Joseph's Middle East Pita Bread (white or whole wheat; lower
   in sodium than other brands)
Joseph's Middle East Soy Pita Bread
Jude's Wheat Pita Bread (whole grain)
Roche Brothers Whole Wheat Pita
Sahara Whole Wheat Pita Bread

Rolls and Buns

Bouyea-Fassetts Cracked Wheat Classic Rolls
Trader Joe's whole wheat hamburger or hot dog buns

Tortillas

Homestyle Kitchens (Tumaro's) Gourmet Tortilla Wraps (for
   burritos)
Maria and Ricardo's Tortillas
Whole Foods Tortillas

BREAKFAST FOODS

Eggs

Eggstro'dnaire Egg Product
Fleischmann's Egg Beaters
Fleischmann's Egg Beaters Vegetable Omelet Mix
Morningstar Farms Scramblers
Second Nature No Cholesterol Egg Product

Pancakes and Waffles

Aunt Jemima Lite Pancake Mix
Aunt Jemima Whole Wheat Pancake Mix
Hungry Jack Buttermilk complete mixes
Kellogg's Special K Waffles (frozen)
Krusteaz Oat Bran Lite Complete Pancake Mix

Sausages

Boca Breakfast Links (sausage flavor, soy)
Boca Breakfast Patties (sausage flavor, soy)
Healthy Choice Low-Fat Breakfast Sausages
Morningstar Farms Breakfast Links (sausage flavor, soy)
Morningstar Farms Breakfast Patties (sausage flavor, soy)
Morningstar Farms Breakfast Strips (bacon flavor, soy)

CAKES, PASTRIES

The following items are high in sugar and should be eaten in moderation.

Drake's Light & Fruity Apple Coffee Cakes
Entenmann's fat-free, cholesterol-free cakes and pastries
"Hostess Lights" Cupcakes
Pillsbury Lovin' Lites brownie mix
"Sara Lee Lights" French Cheesecake
Sara Lee Free & Light Strawberry Yogurt Dessert
Other Sara Lee Free & Light desserts

CEREALS

The following cereals met four or five of the following five criteria for healthy cereals: less than 200 mg of sodium, trans fat free, less than or equal to 5 grams of sugar, greater than or equal to 3 grams of fiber, less than or equal to 160 calories.

Arrowhead Mills Nature O's
Barbara's Crispy Wheats
Barbara's Grain Shop
Barbara's Puffins
Barbara's Shredded Spoonfuls
Barbara's Soy Essence
Cheerios
Cream of wheat
Erewhon instant oatmeal
GM Fiber One
Grainfields Toasted Oats
Grape-Nuts Flakes
Health Valley Blue Corn Flakes
Health Valley Healthy Crunches & Flakes
Health Valley Organic Fiber 7 Multigrain Flakes
Heritage Bites (Nature's Path)
Kamut
Kashi (From Kashi to Good Friends)
Kashi Breakfast Pilaf
Kashi Go Lean
Kashi Heart to Heart
Kashi Medley
Kashi Puffed
Kellogg's All Bran
Kellogg's Bran Buds
Lifestream Flax Plus
Nutlettes Soy Cereal
Post Shredded Wheat N' Bran
President's Choice Ancient Grains
Quaker Oats Old Fashioned Oatmeal
Shredded Wheat
Total (whole-grain)
Uncle Sam

Wheatabix
Wheatena

CHEESES

Preferably any cheese with about 3 grams of fat and 200 mg sodium per ounce
Alpine Lace cheese, fat free or low fat
Alpine Lace Free 'N Lean Fat-Free Party Spread (cream cheese product with garlic and herbs)
Alpine Lace Goat Cheese, 50 percent less fat
Breakstone Dry Curd Cottage Cheese (fat free)
Cabot Cheddar, 75 percent fat free
Cabot Light Vitalait Cheese
Chavrie Goat Cheese
Denmark's Finest Light Havarti
Dragone Lite Cheese—Mozzarella
Finlandia Light Swiss Cheese
Friendship Farmer Cheese
Galaxy Veggie Slices
Healthy Choice Fat Free Cream Cheese
Hood Lite Cottage Cheese, no salt added
Hood Nuform Lowfat Cottage Cheese (99 percent fat free)
Jarlsberg Lite Swiss
King's Choice Light Harvarti Cheese
Kraft Healthy Favorites Fat Free Cheddar
Kraft Light Naturals (Monterey Jack)
Laughing Cow Light Spreadable Cheese
Lifetime Fat Free Cheese
Philadelphia Nonfat Cream Cheese
President Fat Free Feta
Sargento Preferred Light Mozzarella
Smart Beat Fat Free Non-Dairy Cheese
Sorrento Low Fat Mozzarella
Tasty-Lo, by Edam Cheeses
Trader Joe's Reduced Fat Gouda

Weight Watchers Part–Skim Milk Cheese
Wispride Light Soft Port Wine Cheese

COOKIES

BP Gourmet Cookies (very low calorie)
Entenmann's fat-free, cholesterol-free cookies
French Twists or Café Twists
Frookies Fat Free
Frookies Fruitins
Girl Scout Reduced Fat Strawberries n' Creme Cookies
Graham crackers
Greenfield fat-free cookies
Health Valley cookies
Mi-Del Snaps
Nabisco Fig Newtons or any fat-free fruit Newton
Nabisco Honey Maid Cinnamon Grahams
Nabisco Old Fashioned Ginger Snaps
Nabisco Snackwell's products
Santa Fe Farms products
Stouffer's Animal Crackers
Sunshine Golden Fruit Biscuit Cookies
Trader Joe's Meringues

CRACKERS

Bold type indicates whole-grain choices; all products listed are free of or contain minute amounts of trans fats.
Ak-Mak crackers
Barbara's Rite Lite Rounds (similar in taste to Ritz)
Barbara's Wafer Crisps
Barbara's Wheatines
Good Health Quilt Crackers
Health Valley fat-free crackers
Kashi TLC (Tasty Little Crackers)

Kavli Crispbread
Manischewitz Whole Wheat Matzo Crackers
Nabisco Fat-Free Premium crackers
Nabisco Snackwell's crackers
Old London Melba Snacks
Rykrisp
Ryvita
Unsalted Tops Saltines
Wasa Crispbread
Woven Wheats by Whole Foods (similar to Triscuit)

FROZEN DESSERTS

Breyers fat-free and light ice creams
Colombo Shoppe Style Frozen Yogurt
Dole Fruit 'n Yogurt Bars
Dole fruit sorbet
Edy's fat-free ice cream or sugar-free low-fat ice cream
Edy's light ice cream
Elan frozen yogurt
Healthy Choice Frozen Dairy Dessert
Hendries Fudgsicle Fudge Pops
Kemps nonfat frozen yogurt
Lite Tofutti (nondairy frozen dessert)
Sealtest Free nonfat frozen dessert bars
Sealtest Free nonfat frozen yogurt or ice cream
Simple Pleasures frozen dairy dessert
Stonyfield Farm frozen yogurt
Weight Watchers Chocolate Mousse (frozen bars, contain
    NutraSweet)
Weight Watchers fat-free products
To help control portions of frozen desserts, try:
Keebler Ice Cream Cups
Nabisco Comet Cups
Nabisco Comet Sugar Cones

FROZEN DINNERS

Choose entrées with less than 4 grams of saturated fat and 600 mg of sodium per serving. The following brands have many good selections within this range:

Cascadian Farms—Meals for a Small Planet (800-624-4123, if not available in store)

Healthy Choice

Lean Cuisine

Smart Ones

Stouffer's Right Course

Weight Watchers

INGREDIENTS

Baking Ingredients

Carnation Evaporated Skim Milk

Comstock Light Cherry Filling or Topping

Lucky Leaf Lite Cherry Pie Filling (lower sugar content)

Mori-Nu Mates low-fat pudding powder mixes for tofu

Silk Soymilk Creamer

Smuckers Baking Healthy Oil and Shortening Replacement (fat free; the consistency of thick applesauce)

Quaker Unprocessed Bran (wheat bran)

Wonderslim Fat Free Pie Crust

Condiments

Angostura Low Sodium Soy Sauce (62 percent less sodium than soy sauce)

Chi Chi's salsa

Enrico's Salsa, no salt added

KC Masterpiece BBQ sauce (lower in sodium than most brands)

Light 'n Lively Free (nonfat sour cream alternative)

Light tamari sauce

Vinegar

MARGARINES/BUTTERS

Tub margarines/butters preferred over sticks; bold type indicates most recommended.

Benecol Light Spread

Brummel and Brown Yogurt Spread

Fleischmann's Extra Light Margarine

Fleischmann's Lower Fat Margarine

I Can't Believe It's Not Butter—Light

I Can't Believe It's Not Butter—pump spray, fat free

Land O'Lakes Light Whipped Butter

Promise Extra Light (40 percent vegetable oil spread)

Promise Ultra (26 percent vegetable oil spread; look for green package

Promise Ultra Fat Free Spread

Smart Balance Light

Smart Beat Spread, trans fat free

Spectrum Spread, trans fat free

Take Control Spread

Weight Watchers Country Cottage Farms Extra Light Spread

MAYONNAISE

Bright Day Dressing

Cains (fat free or reduced fat)

Hellmann's Dijonnaise (mustard and mayonnaise blend)

Hellmann's Lite

Kraft Free Nonfat Mayonnaise Dressing

Kraft Miracle Whip Free or Kraft Light

Miracle Whip Light (reduced-calorie salad dressing)

Smart Beat Mayonnaise

Weight Watchers reduced-calorie mayonnaise

MEAT, POULTRY, FISH

Bold type indicates no skin ground in.

Banquet Fat Free Baked Breast Patties (frozen)

Banquet Fat Free Baked Breast Tenders (frozen)
Butterball Fat Free Ground Turkey
Butterball Fat Free Polska Kielbasa
Healthy Choice Breaded Fish Sticks
Healthy Choice Extra Lean Low Fat Ground Beef
Healthy Choice Franks
Healthy Choice Low Fat Polska Kielbasa
Hebrew National Beef Franks, 97 percent fat free
Hormel Light & Lean Franks, 97 percent fat free
Jennie-O Turkey Store Ground Turkey
King Oscar Sardines in Water, no salt added
Louis Rich Turkey Breast (roast, slices, steaks, or tenderloin)
Mrs. Paul's Healthy Treasures Breaded Fish Sticks
Mrs. Paul's Light Haddock or Cod
Oscar Mayer Fat Free Hot Dogs
Oscar Mayer Healthy Favorites Hot Dogs (97 percent fat free)
Perdue Lean Ground Turkey
Shady Brook Farms Ground Turkey
Van de Kamp's Crisp & Healthy Baked, Breaded Fish Sticks
    (3 g fat; 97 percent fat free)

PASTA

Be wary of refrigerated pastas because they usually contain eggs.

Hodgson Mill Whole Wheat Pasta
Louise's or Ferrara gnocchi (frozen)
Mama Rosie's Low Fat Cheese Ravioli or Spinach and Cheese
    Ravioli
Mrs. T's Low Fat Frozen Pierogies
No Yolks (no-cholesterol egg noodles)
Prince Healthy Harvest Whole Wheat Blend Pasta
The Original Gourmet Rainbow Cheese Tortellini (lowest-
    saturated-fat cheese tortellini)
Westbrae Natural Whole Wheat Pasta

PEANUT BUTTER

Arrowhead Mills
Maranatha natural nut butters (peanut or almond)
Smucker's Old Fashioned Peanut Butter
Teddie Natural Peanut Butter
Trader Joe's Natural Peanut Butter (smooth or chunky)

SALAD DRESSINGS

Regular, light, or low-fat varieties with a liquid oil (any brand)

SAUCES

Enrico's Tomato Sauce, no salt added
Healthy Choice Spaghetti Sauce
Hunt's Light Spaghetti Sauce (traditional or with mushrooms)
Prego Spaghetti Sauce, no salt added
Ragu Today's Recipe Pasta Sauce

SEASONINGS

Butter substitutes include:
Butter Buds (natural butter-flavored mix—very low in
    sodium)
Molly McButter (has moderate amounts of sodium)
Salt substitutes include:
Cardia
Lawry's Natural Choice seasonings
Mrs. Dash
Nu Salt
Papa Dash Lite Lite Lite Salt (black label)

SNACKS

Chips, Popcorn, etc.

Bearitos tortilla chips
Boston's Lighter Choice Popcorn (green bag)

Cape Cod Potato Chips, 40 percent reduced fat (made with canola oil)
Garden of Eatin' tortilla chips
Good Health Baked Potato Sticks
Healthy Choice Microwave Popcorn
Louise's Caramel Fat Free Popcorn
Louise's low-fat potato chips
Orville Redenbacher's Smart Pop Microwave Popcorn
Pop Secret Microwave Popcorn, 94 percent fat free
Veggie Chips, by Snack Appeal, 95 percent fat free
Vic's Popcorn
Wege Honey Wheat Pretzels

Other

Hains Honey Nut or Apple Cinnamon Mini Rice Cakes
Nature's Choice Real Fruit Bars
Nature Valley Low Fat Granola Bars
Planters Reduced Fat Honey Roasted Peanuts
Snackwell's Cheese Crackers
Stella D'Oro Fat Free Breadsticks
Quaker Fat Free Corn Cakes (caramel corn)

Sauces, Dips

Guiltless Gourmet No-Fat Picante Sauce
Guiltless Gourmet Spicy Black Bean Dip

SOUPS

Bean Cuisine boxed soups
Campbell's Healthy Request products
Fantastic Foods dehydrated cups
Hains fat-free soups
Health Valley fat-free soups
Healthy Choice soups
Herb-Ox Low Sodium Instant Broth and Seasoning (chicken or beef flavor)
Organic Gourmet Low Sodium Vegetable Bouillon

Pritikin soups (vegetable, tomato, or minestrone)
Progresso "Healthy Classics"
Spice Islands dehydrated cups
Westbrae Natural fat-free soups

VEGETARIAN ENTREES AND PROTEIN SOURCES

Beans

Amy's Burritos (soy and bean)
Bush's Vegetarian Baked Beans
Hains Vegetarian Fat Free Baked Beans
Health Valley Fat-Free Chili
Health Valley Mild Vegetarian Chili, no salt added
Old El Paso Fat Free Refried Beans
President's Choice Lentil & Bean Vegetable Patty

Cheese Substitutes

Soya Kaas
Veggie Slices, by Galaxy

Meat Substitutes

Amy's Texas Veggie Burger
Boca Burgers (soy)
Boca Meatless Breakfast Links or Patties (soy)
Boca Meatless Tenders
Boca Sausages—Italian (soy protein)
Fantastic Foods Nature's Burger or Mix (veggies, brown
    rice)
Fantastic Foods Nature's Sausage Mix
Franklin Farms Portabella Burgers
Franklin Farms VeggiBalls (vegetable meatballs)
Gardenburger Veggie Patty or LifeBurger
Health Is Wealth Chicken-Free Nuggets (boxed, frozen)
Heart and Natural Burger (soy)
Knox Mountain Healthy Burger
Lightlife Fat Free Smart Dogs (soy)
Lightlife Lean Italian Links

Lightlife Light Burger (soy)

Lightlife Smart Deli Bologna

Lightlife Smart Ground (meatless crumbles)

Morningstar Farms Breakfast Links (sausage flavor, textured vegetable protein)

Morningstar Farms Breakfast Patties (sausage flavor, textured vegetable protein)

Morningstar Farms Breakfast Strips (bacon flavor, textured vegetable protein)

Morningstar Farms Chik Nuggets or Chik Patties (breaded, baked chicken substitute)

Morningstar Farms Griller Crumbles (ground meat substitute—soy)

Morningstar Farms Meat-Free Buffalo Wings (hot and spicy veggie drumettes)

Morningstar Farms stuffed sandwiches

Morningstar Farms Veggie Burgers (soy)

Natural Touch Okara Pattie

New Menu Vegi-Burger (soy)

New Menu VegiDogs (soy)

Veggie Patch Buffalo Wings (soy)

Veggie Patch Veggitinos (vegetable meatballs)

Yves Soy Protein Deli Slices

Yves Veggie Breakfast Links

Yves Veggie Chili Dogs (soy)

Yves Veggie Ground Round (soy)

Pasta, Pizza, etc.

Bean Cuisine pasta and bean mixes, low-sodium

Farm Foods PizSoy (pizza alternative)

Soy Boy Tofu Ravioli

Terrazza pasta/bean meals (boxed)

Trader Joe's Herbed Tofu Ravioli

Trader Joe's Manicotti Florentine (soy)

Yves Veggie Cuisine Pepperoni

Other

Dixie Diners Crunchy Chocolate Soy Rocks

Edamame (fresh or frozen soybeans; packed either in pod or out)

Fantastic Foods Tofu Scrambler

GeniSoy Soy Protein Bar

Golden Cheese Blintzes, low fat (frozen)

Golden Zucchini Pancakes

Health Source Soy Protein Shake

Health Trip Company Soynut Butter

Nature Valley granola bars

Hummus (Cedars, Mr. Hummus)

Lightlife Savory Seitan (wheat protein source)

Lightlife Tofu Pups (soy)

Miso (soy-based soup)

Mori-Nu Mates low-fat pudding powder mixes for tofu

Nutlettes (soy protein)

Seaside Farms edamame

Smoke & Fire Lemon Garlic Smoked Tofu

Snacking Delight Smart Soy Cookies

Soy beverage, with calcium

Soy Boy 5 Graub Tempeh (refrigerated)

Soy nuts

Soy powders (Challenge, GeniSoy, or Health Source)

Spice Islands Good Harvest side dishes, low sodium (stuffing or potato)

Taverno Classic Spinach Pie (frozen)

Tempeh (soy) (all varieties)

Tofu (soy) (all varieties)

Tofu salad from Bread and Circus (use as egg salad substitute)

Trader Joe's Breaded Soy Patties

Trader Joe's Pad Thai with Tofu

Trader Joe's Roasted Soybean Butter (peanut butter substitute)

Trader Joe's Vegetable Gyoza Potstickers

Tree of Life Smoked Tofu (soy) or Baked Tofu (white wave on package)
Veggie Patch Spinach Veggie Nuggets
West Soy (lite) Non Dairy Soy Beverage (100 percent organic; refrigerate upon opening)
Whole Foods Soy Protein Powder

YOGURT

Columbo Nonfat Lite 100 Yogurt
Dannon Light Yogurt, no fat, no sugar
Dannon nonfat and low-fat yogurts
Horizon Organic Fat Free Yogurt
Silk Soy Yogurt
Stonyfield Farm fat-free yogurts
Stonyfield Farm Yosqueeze, low fat
WholeSoy Soy Yogurt
Yoplait 150 Nonfat Yogurt

MIND/BODY MEDICAL INSTITUTE (GENERAL)

You can order the following audiotapes, videotapes, and CDs directly from the Mind/Body Medical Institute (824 Boylston Street, Chestnut Hill, MA 02467; 617-991-0102 or toll-free, 866-509-0732; tapes and CDs can also be ordered from the website: www.mbmi.org). Please make checks payable to the Mind/Body Medical Institute. No tax or postage is required. You can also visit your local or online bookstore to see what other CDs and tapes may be available.

AUDIOTAPES

All audiotapes are $12.

Body Scan with Ocean Sounds (female voice)
Side 1 (17 minutes) elicits the relaxation response through a slow body scan that has a breath focus. Side 2 (17 minutes) uses ocean sounds and breath awareness to foster relaxation and healing.

Exercise and the Relaxation Response (male voice)
Side 1 (31 minutes) offers instruction on how to elicit the relaxation response while exercising, to enhance your health as you improve your physical fitness. Side 2 (31 minutes) has nondistracting music that helps you maintain a rhythm once you no longer need instruction from side 1.

Basic Relaxation Exercise/Mindfulness Meditation (female voice)
Side 1 (20 minutes) introduces you to the relaxation response, including some key techniques such as breath awareness, body scan relaxation, and use of a focus word. Side 2 (20 minutes) teaches awareness, or "mindfulness," of sensations, thoughts, and sounds.

A Gift of Relaxation/Garden of Your Mind (female voice)
Side 1, "Gift of Relaxation" (20 minutes), introduces the basic steps of eliciting the relaxation response, using a body scan exercise and some simple deep breathing techniques. Side 2, "Garden of Your Mind" (20 minutes), begins with body scan relaxation and breath awareness and then incorporates imagery of a lovely garden, one that you have either visited in your past or that you create in your own mind. Both sides of the tape end with positive affirmations, encouraging you to feel good about yourself and proud of your experience.

Basic Relaxation Response Exercise (male voice)
Side 1 (20 minutes) is similar to the Basic Relaxation Exercise/Mindfulness Meditation tape but also introduces breath awareness and body scan relaxation. Side 2 (45 minutes) includes frequent pauses to allow you to practice the relaxation response.

Advanced Relaxation Response (female voice)
Side 1 (30 minutes) guides you through a body scan as a way to practice the relaxation response. Side 2 (50 minutes) reinforces basic relaxation skills and also guides you through a stretching routine and a series of images for healing.

Self Empathy/Nurturing Change (female voice)
Side 1 (20 minutes) uses music and guided meditation to counter anxiety and to foster progressive body relaxation, plus breath focus to support nonjudging awareness. Side 2 (18 minutes) uses music and guided meditation to enhance self-awareness for greater physical and emotional well-being.

Extended Relaxation Exercise/Beach Walk Mental Imagery
(female voice)
The guidance in this tape is very specific, making it easy to follow. Side 1 (40 minutes) focuses on relaxation exercises, including a long body scan and a visualization exercise. Side 2 (20 minutes)

includes breath and other relaxation exercises, as well as a guided imagery exercise involving a sandy beach on a magnificent summer day. (There are no wave sounds in the background.)

Positive Affirmations and Visualization in Weight Loss
(female voice)
Side 1 (20 minutes) uses music and guided meditation to counter anxiety, plus breath focus to support nonjudging awareness followed by body relaxation. Self-empathy, guided by self-awareness, is the ultimate focus. Side 2 (18 minutes) uses music and guided meditation to enhance self-awareness for greater physical and emotional well-being.

Tuning In to Your Body, Tuning Up Your Mind (female voice)
Side 1 (30 minutes) provides exercises to help you release physical tension, loosen joints, and realign posture. Side 2 (30 minutes) includes special instruction in diaphragmatic breathing and gives guidance for using breath to enhance exercise.

VIDEOTAPES

An Introduction to the Mind/Body Medical Institute with Herbert Benson, M.D.
60 minutes; price: $24.99
Herbert Benson, M.D., introduces the field of mind/body medicine and the work of the Mind/Body Medical Institute. He presents the physiology of the stress response and its counterpart, the relaxation response; a brief overview of the history of mind/body medicine; and the aspects of mind/body medicine that are becoming increasingly common in conventional medicine.

Advanced Tibetan Buddhist Meditation: The Investigations of Herbert Benson, M.D.
25 minutes; price: $24.99
This videotape captures an amazing phenomenon. Monks in the Himalayan mountains who practice an advanced form of medita-

tion are shown generating enough body heat in freezing temperatures to dry icy wet sheets on their naked bodies.

Managing Stress through Humor and Choice with Loretta LaRoche
60 minutes; price: $24.99
Stress humorist LaRoche offers humor to reduce stressful situations and helps viewers use laughter to move worries from sublime to the ridiculous.

Staying Healthy in a Stressful World
Price: $19.99
This videotape contains the premiere episode of *Body & Soul*, the national PBS series on mind, body, and spirit. This segment explores the nature of stress and provides relaxation techniques and other strategies in use at the Mind/Body Medical Institute.

CDs

Sights and Sounds: Relaxation
Price: $10
Pop this CD into your computer and take a "mental coffee break" with three easy-to-follow meditations guaranteed to relax and refresh your spirit. You can use it when you are at your desk feeling burned out, when you are flying or stuck in an airport terminal, or before a presentation, exam, or performance. This CD is interactive and also links to the MBMI website.

Eight Relaxation Response Exercises
Price: $20
This CD includes eight guided relaxation exercises with background music and one music track. Ranging from 7 to 10 minutes in length, these relaxation exercises include breath focus, muscle relaxation, and a beach, mountain, and garden relaxation. Both adults and children have found this CD beneficial as a guide for relaxation during the day or before going to sleep at night. Includes one male and two female voices.

MIND/BODY MEDICAL INSTITUTE AFFILIATES

The Mind/Body Medical Institute has affiliates in many states that offer cardiac wellness programs, as well as programs for dealing with a range of stress-related illnesses or illnesses exacerbated by stress. For information about programs in your area, visit our website: www.mbmi.org.

ORGANIZATIONS THAT CAN HELP

To inquire about cardiac rehabilitation programs in your area, contact any of the following groups:

American Association for Cardiovascular and Pulmonary Rehabilitation
401 North Michigan Ave., Suite 2200
Chicago, IL 60611
312-321-5146
www.aacvpr.org

American Heart Association
7272 Greenville Ave.
Dallas, TX 75231
800-242-8721
www.americanheart.org

American Lung Association
61 Broadway, Sixth Floor
New York, NY 10006
212-315-8700
www.lungusa.org

American Stroke Association
7272 Greenville Ave.
Dallas, TX 75231
888-478-7653
www.StrokeAssociation.org

OTHER HELPFUL ORGANIZATIONS

American Diabetes Association
1660 Duke St.
Alexandria, VA 22314
800-DIABETES for the Diabetes Information and Action Line
www.diabetes.org

American Dietetic Association
216 Jackson Blvd.
Chicago, IL 60606-6995
312-899-0040
www.eatright.org

American Obesity Association
1250 24th St., NW, Suite 300
Washington, DC 20037
800-986-2372
202-776-7712
www.obesity.org

National Cholesterol Education Program
NHLBI Health Information Network
PO Box 30105
Bethesda, MD 20824-0105
301-592-8573
800-575-9355 (consumer hot line with recorded messages)
www.nhlbi.nih.gov

Overeaters Anonymous
6075 Zenith Court NE
Rio Rancho, NM 87124
505-891-2664
www.overeatersanonymous.org

Weight Control Information Network
1 WIN Way
Bethesda, MD 20892-3665
877-946-4627 (toll free)
202-828-1025
www.niddk.nih.gov/health/nutrit/win.htm

SUGGESTED READING

BOOKS

A Sampling of Additional Books by Herbert Benson and MBMI Staff
(Many have been updated or are available in paperback.)

Benson, Herbert. *The Relaxation Response.* New York: Avon
Books, 1975.

———. *Beyond the Relaxation Response: How to Harness the
Healing Power of Your Personal Beliefs.* New York: Times Books,
1984.

———. *Timeless Healing: The Power and Biology of Belief.* New
York: Scribner, 1996.

———. *The Breakout Principle: How to Activate the Natural Trigger
That Maximizes Creativity, Athletic Performance, Productivity
and Personal Well-Being.* New York: Scribner, 2003.

Benson, Herbert, and Eileen Stuart. *The Wellness Book: The
Comprehensive Guide to Maintaining Health and Treating Stress-
Related Illness.* New York: Carol Publishing Group, 1992 (out
of print).

Domar, Alice D., and Henry Dreher. *Healing Mind, Healthy
Woman: Using the Mind-Body Connection to Manage Stress and
Take Control of Your Life.* New York: Dell, 1997.

———. *Self-Nurture: Learning to Care for Yourself as Effectively
as You Care for Everyone Else.* New York: Viking Penguin,
1999.

A Sampling of Useful Books by Other Authors

ANGER

Williams, Redford, and Virginia Williams. *Anger Kills: Seventeen Strategies for Controlling the Hostility That Can Harm Your Health*. New York: Harper Mass Market Paperback, 1998.
———. *Lifeskills: Eight Simple Ways to Build Stronger Relationships, Communicate More Clearly, and Improve Health*. New York: Times Books, 1999.

BUILDING BELIEFS

Frankl, Viktor E. *Man's Search for Meaning*. New York: Washington Square Press, 1997.

Peck, M. Scott. *The Road Less Traveled: A New Psychology of Love, Traditional Values and Spiritual Growth*, 2nd ed. New York: Touchstone Books, 1998.

COGNITIVE RESTRUCTURING

Blanchard, Kenneth, and Spencer Johnson. *The One Minute Manager*. New York: William Morrow and Company, 1982.

Burns, David. *Feeling Good: The New Mood Therapy*. New York: William Morrow and Company, 1980.
———. *The Feeling Good Handbook, Revised*. New York: Plume, 1999.

Carlson, Richard. *Don't Sweat the Small Stuff . . . And It's All Small Stuff*. New York: Hyperion, 1997.
———. *What About the Big Stuff? Finding Strength and Moving Forward when the Stakes Are High*. New York: Hyperion, 2002.

Carlson, Richard, and Joseph Bailey. *Slowing Down the Speed of Life: How to Create a More Peaceful, Simpler Life from the Inside Out*. San Francisco: Harper San Francisco, 1998.

Johnson, Spencer. *Who Moved My Cheese? An Amazing Way to Deal with Change in Your Work and Your Life*. New York: Putnam, 1998.

COPING

Jeffers, Susan. *Feel the Fear and Do It Anyway.* New York:
Harcourt, 1990.

Ornish, Dean. *Love and Survival: Eight Pathways to Intimacy and
Health.* New York: HarperCollins, 1999.

Sinatra, Stephen. *Optimum Health: A Natural Lifesaving
Prescription for Your Body and Mind.* New York: Bantam
Doubleday, 1998.

Sotile, Wayne. *Thriving with Heart Disease.* New York: Free Press,
2003.

DEPRESSION

Styron, William. *Darkness Visible: A Memoir of Madness.* New
York: Random House, 1990.

EXERCISE/YOGA

American College of Sports Medicine. *ACSM Fitness Book,* 3rd
ed. Human Kinetics, 2003.

Anderson, Sandra, and Rolf Sovik, Psy.D. *Yoga: Mastering the
Basics.* Homedale, Pa: Himalayan Institute Press, 2002.

Lynch, Jerry, and Al Chungliang Huang. *Working Out, Working
Within: The Tao on Inner Fitness Through Sports.* New York:
Jeremy P. Tacher/Putnam, 1998.

Scott Kortge, Carolyn. *The Spirited Walker: Fitness Walking for
Clarity, Balance, and Spiritual Connection.* San Francisco:
Harper San Francisco, 1998.

MIND/BODY CONNECTION

Borysenko, Joan. *Guilt Is the Teacher; Love Is the Lesson.* New York:
Warner Books, 1991.

Childre, Doc Lew. *The Heart Math Solution: The Institute of Heart
Math's Revolutionary Program for Engaging the Power of the
Heart's Intelligence.* San Francisco: Harper San Francisco,
1999.

MINDFULNESS

Kabat-Zinn, Jon. *Wherever You Go, There You Are: Mindfulness Meditation in Everyday Life*. New York: Hyperion, 1994.

Nhat Hanh, Thich. *The Miracle of Mindfulness: An Introduction to the Practice of Meditation*. Boston: Beacon Press, 1999.

NUTRITION

Fletcher, Anne, and Jane Brody. *Thin for Life: Ten Keys to Success from People Who Have Lost Weight and Kept It Off*. New York: Houghton Mifflin, 2001.

Heber, D. *What Color Is Your Diet?* New York: HarperCollins, 2001.

Reaven, G. M., T. K. Strom, and B. Fox. *Syndrome X, the Silent Killer: The New Heart Disease Risk*. New York: Fireside, 2001.

Willett, Walter C. *Eat, Drink, and Be Healthy: The Harvard Medical School Guide to Healthy Eating*. New York: Simon & Schuster Source, 2001.

NEWSLETTERS, MAGAZINES

Cooking Light
PO Box 62376
Tampa, FL 33662-3768
800-336-0125
www.cookinglight.com

Harvard Heart Letter
Harvard Health Publications
10 Shattuck St., Suite 612
Boston, MA 02115
www.health.harvard.edu

Mayo Clinic Health Letter
www.mayoclinic.com

Nutrition Action Health Letter
(published by Center for Science in the Public Interest)
1875 Connecticut Ave., NW, Suite 300
Washington, DC 20009
202-332-9110
www.cspinet.org/nah

Runner's World Magazine
(Good articles on nutrition and general fitness)
PO Box 7307
Red Oak, IA 51591-0307
www.runnersworld.com

University of California,
Berkeley, *Wellness Letter*
Subscription Department
PO Box 420148
Palm Coast, FL 32142
386-447-6328
www.berkeleywellness.com

WEBSITES

Harvard Health Publications
www.health.harvard.edu

Centers for Disease Control
and Prevention
Diabetes Home Page
www.cdc.gov/nccdphp/ddt/
    ddthome.htm

Joslin Diabetes Center
www.joslin.harvard.edu

National Institutes of Diabetes
    and Digestive and Kidney
    Diseases
www.niddk.nih.gov

Angina: discomfort or pain in the chest caused by insufficient blood supply to the heart and usually relieved by rest

Antioxidant: a substance in food that helps to protect cells against damage from free radicals

Arrhythmia: abnormal heart rhythm that can produce palpitations and fainting

Artery: a blood vessel that transports blood away from the heart to the rest of the body

Atherosclerosis: disease marked by buildup of fatty deposits in artery walls, causing the artery to narrow and impairing blood flow

Atherosclerotic plaque: a cholesterol-rich deposit on an artery wall

Atrium: one of the two upper chambers of the heart

Blood pressure: the force exerted against the walls of the arteries as your heart pumps blood through your body. Blood pressure is measured by two readings expressed in millimeters of mercury. Systolic blood pressure, the higher of the two numbers, measures the pressure created as the heart contracts; diastolic blood pressure measures force exerted as the heart relaxes.

Body mass index (BMI): An estimate of an individual's relative body composition calculated from his or her height and weight

Calorie: the unit for measuring the amount of energy in food

Catheter: a pliable, fine tube used in medical procedures, including percutaneous transluminal coronary angioplasty (PTCA)

Cholesterol: a fatlike substance, produced by the liver and contained in all food from animal sources, that is an essential component of body cells and a precursor of bile acids and certain hormones

Cognitive restructuring: techniques intended to change the way people perceive or interpret an event, in order to reduce stress

Coronary artery disease: damage to the heart caused by narrowing or blockage of the coronary arteries that supply blood to the heart

Diabetes: Type 1 diabetes (insulin dependent) is a disorder in which the pancreas produces insufficient or no insulin, causing abnormally high glucose levels in the blood. It leads to an accelerated degeneration of small blood vessels. Type 2 diabetes, more common, tends to develop in adulthood and involves decreased sensitivity to the effects of insulin. Both increase the risk for heart disease.

Endothelium: inner lining of the artery wall

Fatty acids: constituents of fats; the essential fatty acids are those that the body cannot make on its own and therefore needs to obtain from dietary sources

Fibrinogen: blood protein essential to clotting process

Free radicals: by-products of energy metabolism; these are highly reactive molecules that can damage cells, leaving them more vulnerable to further changes that can lead to heart disease and cancer

Glucose: the body's chief source of energy, a simple sugar that passes easily from the digestive tract into the bloodstream when you consume carbohydrates

High-density lipoprotein (HDL): a "good" lipoprotein that protects the arteries by transporting cholesterol from body cells to the liver for elimination

Homocysteine: an amino acid that may be a risk factor for heart disease

Hormone: a chemical messenger that creates profound physiological changes and plays a role in stress response as well as relaxation response

Hydrogenation: the addition of hydrogen to a compound—particularly to unsaturated oils or soft fats—to harden them

Hypertension: medical term for high blood pressure

Immune system: the collective name for cells, chemicals, and physical barriers that defend the body against infections and protect against disease, including heart disease

Insulin: an anabolic (growth-promoting) hormone produced by the pancreas; it helps to metabolize glucose, amino acids, and fatty acids and store them in cells

Insulin resistance: a reduced sensitivity to insulin's action, which can contribute to Type 2 diabetes

Ischemia: interruption of blood flow that occurs when a blood vessel becomes narrowed or clogged

Lipids: fats, oils, and waxes that serve as building blocks for cells or as energy sources for the body

Lipoproteins: protein-covered fat particles that enable cholesterol and triglycerides to move easily through the blood. The two main types of lipoprotein are high-density and low-density.

Low-density lipoprotein (LDL): a "bad" lipoprotein that transports cholesterol from the liver to the rest of the body and can cause buildup of plaques in the arteries

Myocardial infarction: medical term for heart attack, which is caused by the blockage of one or more of the coronary arteries

Myocardium: heart muscle

Percutaneous transluminal coronary angioplasty (PTCA): a procedure that involves inserting a catheter into the artery and then inflating a balloon to reopen the artery

Phytochemicals: substances in fruits and vegetables that help protect against heart disease and cancer by boosting the body's natural defenses and by helping to counter the damaging effects of carcinogens and free radicals

Platelets: minute, colorless disks in the blood that are instrumental in blood clotting

Psychoneuroendocrine system: a system that involves the interaction of the nervous system and various stress hormones

Risk factor: a behavior, genetic predisposition, or physiological condition that may increase a person's risk of developing a disease

Thrombus: clot made up of red blood cells, platelets, and clotting factors

Triglyceride: the primary type of fat in the body and in the diet, formed from three fatty-acid molecules and one glycerol molecule

Vasodilator: substance that opens up blood vessels

Ventricles: lower chambers of the heart

Chapter 1—Mind Your Heart

American Heart Association. *2001 Heart and Stroke Statistical Update*. Dallas: American Heart Association, 2000.

Kroenke, K., and A. D. Mangelsdorff. "Common Symptoms in Ambulatory Care: Incidence, Evaluation, Therapy and Outcome." *American Journal of Medicine* 86 (1989): 262–66.

Chapter 2—Risky Business

Frasure-Smith, N., and R. Prince. "The Ischemic Heart Disease Life Stress Monitoring Program: Impact on Mortality." *Psychosomatic Medicine* 47 (1985): 431–45.

Kaufmann, M. W., et al. "Relation Between Myocardial Infarction, Depression, Hostility and Death." *American Heart Journal* 138 (1999): 549–54.

National Heart, Lung and Blood Institute, The Framingham Heart Study, www.framingham.com.

Rosengren, A., et al. "Social Influences and Cardiovascular Risk Factors as Determinants of Plasma Fibrinogen Concentration in a General Population Sample of Middle-Aged Men." *British Medical Journal* 300 (1990): 634–38.

Sleight, P., et al. "Blood Pressure Reduction and Cardiovascular Risk in HOPE Study." *Lancet* 358 (2001): 2130–31.

Vanhoutte, P. M. "Platelet-Derived Serotonin, the Endothelium, and Cardiovascular Disease." *Journal of Cardiovascular Pharmacology* 17; suppl. 5 (1991): S6–S12.

Williams, R. B. "Psychological Factors in Coronary Artery Disease: Epidemiological Evidence." *Circulation* 76; suppl. I (1987): I-117–I-123.

Chapter 3—Learn to Elicit the Relaxation Response

Benson, H. *The Relaxation Response*. New York: Avon Books, 1975.
———. *Timeless Healing: The Power and Biology of Belief*. New York: Scribner, 1996.

Hoffman, J. W., et al. "Reduced Sympathetic Nervous System Responsivity Associated with the Relaxation Response." *Science* 215 (1982): 190–92.

Soufer, R., and A. Chekerdjiev. "Stress: From the Aroused Brain to the Reacting Heart." *Cerebrum: The Dana Forum on Brain Science* (winter 2002): 67–78. New York: The Charles A. Dana Foundation, 2002.

Stefano, G. B., G. L. Fricchione, B. T. Slingsby, and H. Benson. "The Placebo Effect and the Relaxation Response: Neural Processes and Their Coupling to Constitutive Nitric Oxide." *Brain Research Reviews* 35 (2001): 1–19.

Chapter 4—Manage Your Stress

Benson, Herbert, and Eileen Stuart. *The Wellness Book: The Comprehensive Guide to Maintaining Health and Treating Stress-Related Illness*. New York: Carol Publishing Group, 1992 (out of print).

Burns, D. *Feeling Good: The New Mood Therapy*. New York: New American Library, 1990.

Ellis, A., and R. Grieger. *Handbook of Rational-Emotive Therapy*, vol. 2. New York: Springer Publishing Co., 1986.

Chapter 5—Dealing with Emotions

Pennebaker, J. W. "Writing Your Wrongs." *American Health* (January–February 1991): 64–67. Adapted from Pennebaker, J. W., *Opening Up: The Healing Power of Confiding in Others* (New York: William Morrow, 1990).

Pennebaker, J. W., and J. D. Seagal. "Forming a Story: The Health Benefits of Narrative." *Journal of Clinical Psychology* 55 (1999): 1243–54.

Chapter 6—Balance Your Plate, Help Your Heart

Anderson, J. W., B. M. Johnstone, and M. E. Cook-Newell. "Meta-Analysis of the Effects of Soy Protein Intake on Serum Lipids." *New England Journal of Medicine* 333 (1995): 276–82.

Barr, S. L., et al. "Reducing Total Fat without Reducing Saturated Fatty Acids Does Not Significantly Lower Total Plasma Cholesterol Concentrations in Normal Males." *American Journal of Clinical Nutrition* 55 (1992): 675–81.

Burr, M. L., et al. "Effects of Changes in Fat, Fish, and Fiber Intakes on Death and Myocardial Reinfarction: Diet and Reinfarction Trial (DART). *Lancet* 2 (1989): 757–61.

Despres, J. P. "Hyperinsulinemia as an Independent Risk Factor for Ischemic Heart Disease." *New England Journal of Medicine* 334 (1996): 952–57.

Hodish, I., et al. "Effect of Elevated Homocysteine Levels on Clinical Restenosis following Percutaneous Coronary Intervention." *Cardiology* 97 (2002): 214–17.

Hu, F. B., et al. "Fish and Omega-3 Fatty Acid Intake and Risk of Coronary Heart Disease in Women." *Journal of the American Medical Association* 287 (2002): 1815–21.

National Heart, Lung, and Blood Institute. *Third Report of the National Cholesterol Education Program Expert Panel on Detection, Evaluation, and Treatment of High Blood Cholesterol in Adults,* May 2001.

Sacks, F. M., et al. (DASH-Sodium Collaborative Research Group). "Effects on Blood Pressure of Reduced Dietary Sodium and the Dietary Approaches to Stop Hypertension (DASH) Diet." *New England Journal of Medicine* 344 (2001): 3–10.

Yip, J., et al. "Resistance to Insulin-Mediated Glucose Disposal as a Predictor of Cardiovascular Disease." *Journal of Clinical Endocrinology Metabolism* 83 (1998): 2773–76.

Chapter 7—Improve Your Relationship with Food

Foster, G. D., et al. "What Is a Reasonable Weight Loss? Patients' Expectations and Evaluations of Obesity Treatment Outcomes." *Journal of Consulting Clinical Psychology* 99 (1997): 79–85.

Harnack, L., et al. "Soft Drink Consumption among U.S. Children and Adolescents: Nutritional Consequences." *Journal of the American Dietetic Association* 99 (1999): 436–41.

Mattes, R. D. "Dietary Compensation by Humans for Supplemental Energy Provided as Ethanol or Carbohydrate in Fluids." *Physiology of Behavior* (January 1996): 179–87.

National Heart, Lung, and Blood Institute. *Clinical Guidelines on the Identification, Evaluation, and Treatment of Overweight and Obesity in Adults,* released June 17, 1998.

U.S. Department of Health and Human Services. *The Surgeon General's Call to Action to Prevent and Decrease Overweight and Obesity.* Washington, D.C.: U.S. Department of Health and Human Services, December 2001.

———. *Physical Activity Fundamental to Preventing Disease,* June 20, 2002.

Chapter 8—Exercise Body and Soul

Blair, S. N., et al. "Influences of Cardiorespiratory Fitness and Other Precursors on Cardiovascular Disease and All-Cause Mortality in Men and Women." *Journal of the American Medical Association* 276 (1996): 205–11.

Blumenthal, J. A., et al. "Exercise Treatment for Major Depression: Maintenance of Therapeutic Benefit at 10 Months." *Psychosomatic Medicine* 62 (2000): 633–38.

Haskell, W. L., et al. "Cardiovascular Benefits and Assessment of Physical Activity and Physical Fitness in Adults." *Medicine and Science in Sports and Exercise;* suppl. 24 (1992): S201–S220.

Huddleston, J. S. "Exercise." In *Health Promotion throughout the*

Lifespan, 5th ed., eds. C. Edelman and C. Mandle. Mosby-Yearbook, 2002.

National Institutes of Health Consensus Development Panel on Physical Activity and Cardiovascular Health. "Physical Activity and Cardiovascular Health." *Journal of the American Medical Association* 276 (1996): 241–46.

Pate, R. R., et al. "Physical Activity and Public Health: A Recommendation from the Centers for Disease Control and Prevention and the American College of Sports Medicine." *Journal of the American Medical Association* 273 (1995): 402–7.

Poehlman, E. T., et al. "Physiological Predictors of Increasing Total and Central Adiposity in Aging Men and Women." *Archives of Internal Medicine* 155 (1995): 2443–48.

U.S. Department of Health and Human Services. *Physical Activity and Health: A Report of the Surgeon General.* Washington, D.C.: U.S. Department of Health and Human Services, 1996.

———. *The Surgeon General's Call to Action to Prevent and Decrease Overweight and Obesity.* Washington, D.C.: U.S. Department of Health and Human Services, December 2001.

Williford, H. N., et al. "Exercise Prescription for Women." *Sports Medicine* 15 (1993): 299–311.

Chapter 9—Making It Work

Marlatt, G. A., and J. R. Gordon, eds. *Relapse Prevention: Maintenance Strategies in the Treatment of Addictive Behaviors.* New York: Guilford Press, 1985.

Prochaska, J. O., J. Norcross, and C. DiClemente. *Changing for Good.* New York: Avon Books, 1995.

Unless otherwise noted, all art and tables are provided courtesy of the Mind/Body Medical Institute and Harvard Health Publications.

Unless otherwise noted, all visualization exercises are provided by the Mind/Body Medical Institute.

Chapter 1
Graphic in figure 3 adapted from Barbieri, R. L., A. D. Domar, and K. R. Loughlin, *Six Steps to Increased Fertility* (New York: Simon & Schuster, 2000), 105.

Chapter 2
Art in figure 5 is adapted from Clayman, C. B., ed., *American Medical Association Encyclopedia* (New York: Random House, 1989), 514.

Sidebar 6 is adapted from American Psychiatric Association, "Criteria for Major Depressive Episode," *Diagnostic and Statistical Manual of Mental Disorders*, 4th ed. (Washington, D.C., 1994), 327.

Sidebar 7 is adapted from DiClemente, C. C., and J. O. Prochaska, "Self-Change and Therapy Change of Smoking Behavior: A Comparison of Processes of Change in Cessation and Maintenance," *Addictive Behaviors* 7 (1982): 133–42.

Chapter 3
Sun salute is adapted from Simon, R., and R. Aleskowsky, *Repetitive Strain Injury Handbook* (New York: Henry Holt & Co., 2000).

Art in figures 13 through 18 are adapted from Benson, H., and E. Stuart, *The Wellness Book* (New York: Carol Publishing Group, 1992 [out of print]).

Chapter 4
Table 5 is adapted from Holmes, T. H., and R. H. Rahe, "The Social Readjustment Rating Scale," *Journal of Psychosomatic Research* 11, no. 2 (August 1967): 213–18.

Categories of cognitive distortions are based primarily on the work of Burns, D., *Feeling Good: The New Mood Therapy* (New York: New American Library, 1990). Ellis, A., and R. Grieger, *Handbook of Rational-Emotive Therapy*, vol. 2 (New York: Springer Publishing Co., 1986).

Sidebar 18 has been modified from a Zen koan by the Mind/Body Medical Institute.

Figure 19 is adapted from a drawing by Jim Cassidy.

Chapter 5

Art in Table 10 is based on a model proposed in Kübler-Ross, E., *On Death and Dying* (New York: Scribner, 1997 [reprint]).

Chapter 6

Art in figure 23 is adapted from Heber, D., *What Color Is Your Diet?* (New York: HarperCollins, 2001), 42.

Chapter 8

Sidebar 38, "The Gift of Exercise," was previously published in Huddleston, J. S., "Exercise," in *Health Promotion throughout the Lifespan*, 5th ed., eds. C. Edelman and C. Mandle (Mosby-Yearbook, 2000), 281.

Sidebar 39: The phrase *enlightening the dumbbells* is adapted from a subhead in Douillard, J., *Body, Mind, and Sport: The Mind/Body Guide to Lifelong Fitness and Your Personal Best* (Harmony Books, 1994; or Three Rivers Press (pbk), 2001), 207.

Table 22 is adapted from Karvonen, M., "The Effects of Training Heart Rate: A Longitudinal Study," *Experimental Biology* 35 (1957): 307–15.

Table 23 is adapted from Borg, G. A., "Psychophysical Basis of Perceived Exertion," *Medicine and Science in Sports and Exercise* 14 (1982): 377.

Sidebar 46: Prayers reprinted with permission from Mundy, L., *The Complete Guide to Prayer Walking* (New York: Cross Road Publishers, 1996), chapter 3.

Appendix 1

Recipes for Tempting Tempeh Stir-Fry, Bean Burritos, Cottage by the Cheese, and Yogurt Pie courtesy of Marc O'Meara.

Black Beauty recipe courtesy of Center for Science in the Public Interest.

Muesli and Smoothie recipes courtesy of Food and Health Communications.

AGGIE CASEY, M.S., R.N., is the Director and Clinical Nurse Specialist for the Cardiac Wellness Program. She is also a Researcher and the Clinical Director of Affiliate Cardiac Programs at the Mind/Body Medical Institute; and an Associate in Medicine, Harvard Medical School.

HERBERT BENSON, M.D., is the founding President of the Mind/Body Medical Institute and the Mind/Body Medical Institute Associate Professor of Medicine, Harvard Medical School. A pioneer in mind/body medicine, he defined the relaxation response and continues to lead teaching and research into its efficacy in counteracting the harmful effects of stress.